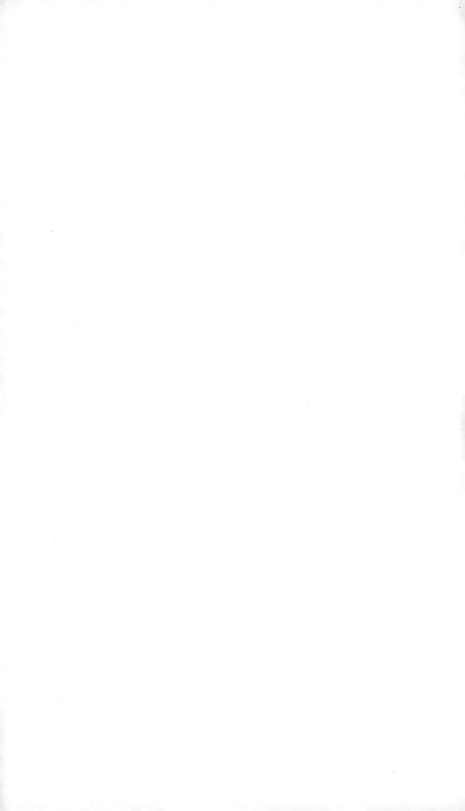

Fat, Stressed, and Sick

Fat, Stressed, and Sick

MSG, Processed Food, and America's Health Crisis

Katherine Reid, PhD
with Barbara Price, PhD

ROWMAN & LITTLEFIELD
Lanham • Boulder • New York • London

This book is not meant to diagnose any condition or replace the advice of the reader's own physician or a trained medical professional. The authors and publisher disclaim any liability or loss that results from the use of information contained within this book.

Published by Rowman & Littlefield
An imprint of The Rowman & Littlefield Publishing Group, Inc.
4501 Forbes Boulevard, Suite 200, Lanham, Maryland 20706
www.rowman.com

86-90 Paul Street, London EC2A 4NE

British Library Cataloguing in Publication Information Available

Library of Congress Cataloging-in-Publication Data

978-1-5381-8076-1 (cloth)
978-1-5381-8077-8 (electronic)

♾™ The paper used in this publication meets the minimum requirements of American National Standard for Information Sciences—Permanence of Paper for Printed Library Materials, ANSI/NISO Z39.48-1992.

I dedicate this book to my children for their love and understanding, and to my incredible clients who have provided the invaluable insights and wisdom that has made this book possible.   —KR

For Lisa and Joshua, who made connecting the dots personal for me.   —BP

CONTENTS

PREFACE

IT'S REMARKABLE HOW MANY SCIENTIFIC DISCOVERIES HAPPEN BY chance. The celebrated science fiction writer and biochemist Isaac Asimov once said, "The most exciting phrase to hear in science, the one that heralds new discoveries, is not 'Eureka!' but 'That's funny....'" You might say chance is how this book came about. A puzzling statement by a parent in an autism chat group spurred Katie Reid to discover the relationship between diet and her daughter's autism symptoms. A keen observer, she took seemingly unrelated events and offhand comments by strangers and formed a hypothesis that, on the face of it, seemed preposterous: her daughter's autism symptoms could be managed by removing glutamate from her diet. Katie also happened to be a biochemist, so she did the research, meticulously connecting the dots. She learned not only that this was true but also that the unprecedented amount of monosodium glutamate that has entered the food supply since the 1970s, primarily in the form of processed food, was likely a factor fueling America's current health crisis.

My involvement with this book also came about by chance, born of an unlikely encounter I had with Katie's husband, Mitch. I was on a private road in the Santa Cruz Mountains, hiking up the mountain with my dog while Mitch was hiking down. In the way that strangers meeting under such circumstances may casually exchange pleasantries, Mitch and I stopped briefly and chatted. That led to meeting Katie and the start of our collaboration.

Since working with Katie on this book, I've come to look at food differently. Now when I walk through the grocery aisles and see the towering shelves of plastic-wrapped, boxed, dehydrated, canned, and processed food, the contents of the neat packages seem more like the sterile residue of something that was once living, as opposed to something you might actually want to eat. These days one may even wonder if what is presented as food has *any* connection to something that was once alive. In the age of manufactured food, what we eat can be made in a lab, constructed from a batch of chemicals and ingredients that are molded into a form and laced with additives scientifically formulated to make you come back for more. If this seems rather dark, well, what a relief it is to stroll the fresh produce aisles! Fruits and vegetables are immediately recognizable in all their shapes and sizes and colors and smells. They are covered by their own skin, veined, stemmed, sunkissed, some even with parts of the earth still clinging to them. I truly did not appreciate the raw, living beauty of whole foods or their profound health benefits until Katie explained it to me.

So when I think about the circumstances and the role that chance played in creating this book, the odd synchronicity of events that led a mom who happened to be a biochemist to discover a way to help her ill daughter (and ultimately define her own life mission), that resulted in a bona fide science writer and editor to show up on the scene just when needed, I feel that it was not just a matter of connecting the dots but having the stars themselves align.

—Barbara Price

INTRODUCTION

December 2005

At the age of 37, I discovered I was pregnant. My husband Mitch and I already had four children (two each from our first marriages) and he was worried about how we were going to manage with yet another. He said having another child now felt like "catching a bowling ball while treading water," a rather dark analogy, I thought. Mitch had recently returned to school to earn a master's degree in business administration and reboot his career in biotechnology. I was working in biotech, too, but I felt that we could manage five children. I did not know what was in store for us.

If you have never had a sibling or a child with special needs, what I am going to describe in the following pages will give you insight into the challenges facing those of us who do. The intractable nature of many childhood illnesses, be it autism, attention deficit hyperactivity disorder (ADHD), psychiatric disorders, even pediatric obesity, is frustrating and heartbreaking. Although this story starts with my grappling with my daughter's autism diagnosis, the lessons I learned are applicable to a wide range of health issues facing families today. And make no mistake: there is an epidemic of childhood disorders impacting our schools, our healthcare system, and the hearts and hopes of families across America.

As a mother and a scientist, I have come to understand that the underlying cause of so many diseases is inflammation, and that inflammation can be managed with a significant change in diet. Specifically, a diet low in free glutamate, commonly referred to as monosodium glutamate or MSG. Despite the messaging from food manufacturers, the idea that serious illnesses are caused by excess glutamate in the diet has been a concern voiced by some members of the medical and scientific community for decades. Here I am not talking about the MSG you sprinkle on your plate at home, but the staggering amount of glutamate that has entered the food supply through the manufacturing of processed food. Once I understood that, our family eliminated processed foods and embraced a diet of whole foods. This has proven so effective in managing my daughter's symptoms that she lost her autism diagnosis.

This book explains the science that shows how reducing the amount of glutamate in your diet can increase your resiliency to disease and help you better manage chronic health issues for everyone in your family.

But before we go there, let me tell you how it began.

August 2006

Our daughter Taylor was born on August 23, 2006, at Stanford Hospital in California. My induced labor and Taylor's birth were uneventful. At home, my mother and my 13-year-old daughter Alice were wonderful care providers. Mitch was less enamored with the baby stage, but he expressed his feelings for his "little girl" in other sweet ways (that didn't involve diaper changes). Yet, around the time Taylor was 18 months old, Mitch began to comment that he didn't feel "bonded" with Taylor. "She doesn't respond to me," he'd say. "She's not affectionate." My typical response was something along the lines of "you just don't spend enough time with her." I, on the other hand, felt very connected to Taylor and so I was quick to dismiss Mitch's concerns.

Taylor, however, did exhibit some odd behaviors that I had not encountered with the older children. About the same time Mitch was voicing his concerns, I became aware of Taylor's insistence on certain routines. For example, when we went for a walk around our neighborhood, we had to take the same path every day. I remember one day I wanted to go on a longer walk than usual and pushed the stroller past our usual turn. Taylor immediately became fussy. As I forged ahead, she screamed and arched her back, trying her best to get out of the seat belt. I stopped the stroller and attempted to calm her again, but to no avail. She writhed and screamed for the next 15 minutes—a most unpleasant walk. As soon as I reached the house, she stopped crying. I let her out of the stroller and she toddled away as if nothing out of the ordinary had happened. I wondered what in the world that was all about. The next day I tried again, and other days as well, but each time I veered from the route, she became distraught. To maintain peace, I stopped trying to forge new paths with Taylor in the stroller.

Similar odd behaviors occurred while she "played" with toys. She had an assortment of plastic animal figures. She didn't arrange them in a typical barnyard scene, such as a pig next to the water trough or a cow next to another cow. She instead lined them up in one big row with the exact same spacing between each animal. My son Mark, who was almost 12 at the time, thought the lineup of the animals was amusing. I recall him picking up the sheep, placing it outside the row, and making a "baa" sound. Taylor didn't see him pick up the sheep, but when she turned around, she immediately picked up the sheep and carefully put it back in the exact same location in the lineup. Mark then moved the cow out of the lineup. This time she saw him move it. Mark playfully made the "moo" sound as he walked the cow around the play area. Instead of engaging in play with her brother, she threw herself on the floor and had a tantrum. Mark and I looked at each other in amazement—her reaction seemed way over the top. During her tantrum, she knocked down most of the toy animals, which caused her to scream more. I decided to ignore the tantrum and walked away. When I returned, she was resetting the animals, all in the exact same order.

When Taylor was between one and a half and two years of age, she began to lag noticeably behind developmental norms. Her language development was slow, but more troubling was her nonverbal communication—or I should say, the lack of it. She didn't point to things she wanted or turn her head when we called her name. At Taylor's 18-month check-up, I mentioned my concerns to the pediatrician. I was told that she was within the normal range in language, albeit on the low side of that range. The evaluation was based on how many words Taylor used. While it was true that she spoke, most of her "words" were animal sounds like "meow" that served no purpose in communicating to us her needs or wants.

3

At Taylor's 24-month appointment, the pediatrician once again dismissed our concerns about her slow language development. I tried to explain that Taylor seemed to be in her own little world, unaware of us or her surroundings, but I didn't get far. Nowhere on the developmental questionnaire was there a checkbox for "she doesn't engage with us."

Shortly after Taylor's second birthday, Mitch told me, "When I hold Taylor in the shower, she rarely makes eye contact with me. If she does, she doesn't hold my gaze." Mitch's experience had been very different when his two older children were toddlers. This was the first time Mitch used the word "autistic" in reference to Taylor. The protective mother in me vaulted to a defensive response: "She's not autistic. She just doesn't like to look at you."

Looking back, I realize I was in denial. There was something different about Taylor, but I reasoned that Taylor had her peculiarities, granted, but what child doesn't? Taylor needed so much more of me, and so everyone else got that much less. The time and attention Taylor needed placed a lot of stress on my relationship with Mitch. I knew Taylor was a major adjustment for everyone, and I desperately wanted everything to be okay. I wanted to convince the family that there was enough love and attention for everyone, and *we* were all okay. As it turned out, it would be a long time before that was true.

November 2009

Taylor was ultimately diagnosed with autism when she was three years old. I now understand that the events leading up to that diagnosis are not unlike those experienced by countless families with a kid on the spectrum: Taylor displayed disruptive behaviors such as grabbing things from other children at preschool and rushing to the classroom door to escape. She failed to recognize social rules such as standing in line for a turn on a slide. She had no interest in activities with other children—it was as if they didn't exist. She had an extreme yet unpredictable sensitivity to some sounds, which elicited loud outbursts at inappropriate times. She also exhibited what we came to call the dreaded yes/no loops. These happened when Taylor wanted something to happen, and at the same time she didn't want it to happen. As a parent, you know that no one can win that one. For example, when washing up before bedtime, she would demand of whoever was helping her that the water faucet be turned off. Then she would demand that it be turned on. Then off, and then on, and so on, becoming more and more distraught. She would end up hysterical, sobbing, "Water on!" "Water off!" "No, on!", unable to stop and walk away from the sink until she was physically lifted and carried to bed. I was quickly becoming overwhelmed, and so I scheduled an appointment with Taylor's pediatrician.

At her appointment, I rattled off a list of Taylor's behaviors. The doctor agreed that these symptoms might be consistent with autism. He told me that I should contact a psychologist for an evaluation. With a diagnosis, Taylor would become eligible for services. I was devastated. There was something about having a medical doctor agree that Taylor could be autistic that crushed my unacknowledged hope that I had it all wrong—somehow, I still harbored hope that my baby was okay. I got into my car and cried. I had no idea what I was supposed to do to support my little girl. I called my sister in tears, telling her that "my little girl's brain seems broken, and I don't know how to fix it."

We met with the psychologist for two 2-hour sessions. The first session was at a local park to allow the psychologist to see how Taylor interacted with other children. The psychologist had brought an assortment of toys, which quickly attracted the attention of perhaps a half-dozen kids. Taylor reacted by abruptly darting away, running about 100 feet up a nearby hill, getting as far away from everyone as she could. She didn't seem upset, just disinterested. We could not coax her back to the play area.

The second session took place in the psychologist's office. The psychologist wanted to see whether Taylor would sing along with her. As soon as the psychologist started singing the nursery rhyme "Mary Had a Little Lamb," Taylor lunged at her, screaming "No! No! No!" I quickly grabbed Taylor, and she calmed down as soon as the psychologist stopped singing. The psychologist then asked Taylor to take off her shoes, which I thought was an odd request at the time. Taylor was more than eager and proceeded to walk on her tippy toes for the remainder of the session. This is a behavior I now understand is associated with autism. When asked to place toys "on top of the chair" or "under the desk," Taylor was not able to follow the instructions. After completing her observations, the psychologist told us she would contact us in a few weeks after she completed a report summarizing the evaluation.

December 2009

Prior to delivering her formal report to the school district, the psychologist came to our home to communicate her assessment. Taylor and I were home alone at the time. I felt my anxiety increase as the psychologist carefully explained her methodology and her observations. She concluded with her diagnosis: "autism, moderate on the spectrum." I thought I was prepared for the diagnosis, but panic gripped me, quickly followed by an overwhelming sense of guilt due to what she said next.

When the psychologist arrived, I'd set Taylor up with a big puzzle, an activity I could count on occupying her so that the psychologist and I could talk. Taylor's play quickly became repetitive, and for the next 10 minutes she inserted and removed the same puzzle piece over and over. Just after rendering her diagnosis, the psychologist then swiveled and pointed at Taylor. Taylor should not be allowed to continue such repetitive play, she said. "Break the cycle." She stated that Taylor needed as many social play opportunities as possible, and that her day should not just be consumed with academic activities like arranging numbers or working on puzzles. The psychologist concluded that Taylor "showed severe to moderate impairment in the area of social interaction" and that this deficit should be promptly addressed.

Making matters worse, she pointed out that she felt I had minimized the seriousness of Taylor's behaviors when we initially spoke on the phone. "Don't take this lightly," she said. "You need to act now." "Act how?" I wondered. "What the heck am I supposed to do now?" Now that we had a diagnosis, I had no idea what our next steps should be. How would I increase social interactions, when we rarely went outside the house without Taylor having some sort of major tantrum? How was I going to encourage social play when every noise upset her?

The psychologist gave us some ideas of possible therapies to explore, and over the course of weeks and months we tried them all. At the time, though, I was completely demoralized. I felt judged. Not only was I *not* doing the "right" things for my child; apparently, I was doing some things wrong.

My family was at the peak of its crisis. The mental and physical drain from caring for Taylor and trying to find help, as her special needs became more apparent, exhausted all of us. The older kids didn't want to invite their friends over to socialize, so they went to their friends' houses instead. At home, I became so attuned to the first sign of repetitious behavior that I would stop whatever I was doing and scurry across the room to redirect Taylor's attention. It felt like our already tenuous family bonds were further disintegrating. Indeed, Taylor's incessant crying and yes/no loops came close to breaking our family apart. Dinners were complete chaos. Mitch and I were frequently angry with each other. His patience was diminishing rapidly, and to make matters worse, Mitch and I were at odds as to how we should intervene. When he observed the yes/no loop, he wanted to send her to her room until she could calm herself. I wanted to distract her or try to soothe her using a gentle voice. In truth, neither approach worked. Mitch and I were desperate and not at all on the same page.

This was the state of affairs when Taylor was diagnosed. She now was eligible for services, and through the Family and Medical Leave Act (FMLA), I was granted one day off a week (for six weeks) to work out Taylor's evaluations, services, health plan, and schedule. I wasn't satisfied with simply arranging for services, however. I was desperate to understand what was happening to my daughter, and I set about to learn everything I could about autism. I became obsessed with reading and learning about brain chemistry, trying to associate her various symptoms to any factor in her environment. Brain biochemistry became my mental retreat from a world that was not making any sense. I asked: What happens in the brain to produce autistic behaviors? More importantly, can the brain change in such a way such that these behaviors are reduced?

I read book after book on the brain, starting with ones that are easier to read, such as *My Stroke of Insight* by Jill Bolte Taylor, and *The Brain That Changes Itself* by Norman Doidge.[1] These books provided me with a new perspective by illustrating that the brain has an amazing capacity to change with its environment. That gave me hope. I also found suggestions in the scientific literature that made me think that food might play a significant role in the brain's functioning. I decided that diet was worth looking into. As Taylor's mom, I could control what Taylor ate, and I could start immediately.

I began researching nutritional deficiencies and how they might affect the brain. Nutrition books, such as *The UltraMind Solution* by Mark Hyman,[2] quickly impressed on me the importance of nutrients for optimal brain function. I learned that autism spectrum disorder (ASD) includes wide-ranging symptoms and is considered a "pervasive disorder" because of its impact on so many systems in the body. Was it possible that diet might be responsible for all of Taylor's pervasive dysfunction? I had my doubts. Nevertheless, I began experimenting with Taylor's diet.

Many children on the autism spectrum have very narrow or self-restricted food preferences. This was certainly the case with Taylor. She would often insist on specific foods, and if she didn't get those foods, a meltdown would invariably ensue. With so many battles, I often gave in, selecting foods that would elicit the least objection and minimize the conflict. Taylor was very much into her routine of bagel and cream cheese in the morning, and she frequently begged for pizza for dinner. A green vegetable was served at most lunches and dinners, but in fact few greens were actually consumed.

I initially supplemented Taylor's diet with specific nutrients that are common deficiencies in SAD—the Standard American Diet. These supplements included magnesium, omega 3s, vitamin D3, and vitamin B complex. I also supplemented her diet with a probiotic. However, before you go out and purchase these supplements, please read on about why and how these were ultimately replaced. You should also know that I define "deficiency" more broadly than most. The recommended daily allowance (RDA), for example, is defined as "the average amount of a nutrient necessary to avoid onset of chronic disease." In my view, deficiency means any level lower than what's needed for optimal health, not just the level needed to prevent chronic disease. We need to thrive, not merely survive!

Getting supplements into Taylor, now three and a half years old, proved to be quite a challenge. She couldn't swallow pills, and I couldn't find a single chewable or liquid form of a supplement that didn't have all sorts of potentially harmful additives. I solved the problem by grinding solid pill supplements in a coffee grinder and mixing them in a blender with raw—and whenever possible, organic—whole foods, such as vegetables, herbs, nuts, seeds, and fruits. We nicknamed this blended concoction our "smoothie," and a routine was born.

Initially, Taylor and I were the only family members consuming smoothies, and Taylor was, shall I say, a highly persuaded participant. I started to feel significantly more energetic throughout the day and mentally noted that I was only consuming the smoothie, not the supplements. I also saw improvements in Taylor. While this next sentence sounds like hyperbole, it is not. Within a week of beginning her smoothie/supplements regimen, Taylor started making eye contact with me. She appeared more responsive to her own name, and she seemed to be more interested in communicating with others. These small changes were my first indication that improvements were possible, and even these small changes gave me a glimmer of hope.

During this period, I called my aunt to give her an update on Taylor, and I quipped about our next "Taylor experiment." She was a bit horrified, saying, "Well, of course you don't mean you are experimenting on Taylor!" Indeed, we were experimenting. With autism, everyone is experimenting.

Seeing Taylor's behavior improve, even marginally, in response to the nutrient-rich smoothies put me squarely on the path of investigating the effects of diet on the brain. As I continued to research this topic, I encountered many internet postings about a gluten-free/casein-free (GC/CF) diet that was claimed to help autistic symptoms. However, then—as is still the case now—clinical studies on the effect of diet on autism were scarce, making it extremely challenging to figure out our next steps. However, on the strength of the anecdotal accounts I read online, I decided to try the GF/CF diet. I started Taylor on the diet about three weeks after starting the smoothie routine. Implementing such a drastic dietary change—especially so close to the winter holiday—was challenging. Cooking our traditional holiday foods was out of the question. Simply figuring out what foods contained gluten and casein took some time and detective work. Fortunately, grocers and food manufacturers had begun labeling items as gluten-free and casein-free. (This was not the godsend I thought it was at the time. It turns out that the processing necessary to remove gluten and casein from foods creates problems, as you will see explained later in this book.)

When I first heard about the GF/CF diet, I wasn't even sure what gluten and casein were, exactly. I learned that gluten is composed of large proteins found in grains such as wheat, barley, and rye. Casein is a class of proteins found in all dairy products. At first, I did not understand the connection between these proteins and why removing them from a person's diet might offer health benefits. It took me another six months to generate a scientific hypothesis connecting these specific proteins to the variety of effects people experience when they stop consuming them. For now, I'll simply point out that both gluten and casein contain very high amounts of the amino acid glutamic acid (also known as glutamate), one of twenty common amino acids found in proteins.

January 2010

After about five weeks on the GF/CF diet, with some trial and error involved, we began to see further improvement in Taylor's behaviors. She started to show interest in socializing with other children, although her social boundaries were ill-defined and often inappropriate. Taylor's ability to communicate improved, too. Whereas previously she hadn't used any words or gestures to communicate her needs, she started using simple one- or two-word sentences. She couldn't engage in conversation, though. For example, when asked questions like "What is your favorite color?" there was still no response. While overall she seemed calmer, things in her environment—such as certain sounds—continued to make her fearful. Changes to her routine still increased her anxiety. Some of the repetitive behaviors, like stacking blocks over and over again, were less frequent but still present, and the yes/no loop continued.

So, while there were noticeable improvements on the GF/CF diet, many of Taylor's autistic traits persisted. I continued to search for additional therapies from healthcare professionals that might help Taylor. We tried a slew of different approaches, including applied behavior analysis (ABA), starting Taylor in a special needs school, speech therapy, and auditory integration therapy (AIT).

April 2010

In the midst of AIT therapy, special needs school three days a week, a new nanny, the GF/CF diet, speech therapy once a week, and gymnastics (more for social interaction than for athletic development), I found myself consumed by a schedule I myself had designed in an attempt to meet Taylor's needs. I was working full time and commuting in ever-increasing traffic in the San Francisco Bay Area. Mitch kept his distance, spending time with Taylor on his terms. The older kids were at an age when they were trying to evade parental controls and were increasingly relieved to have me preoccupied with anything that was not them. And despite all our efforts to meet Taylor's needs, I felt like she had hit a plateau. The fledgling optimism I felt after changing the diet started to recede, and in my worst days, I felt frighteningly close to imagining that the "plateau" I was seeing was actually as far as she would ever go.

At this point, I stepped back and tried to think like a scientist. What was working? What was not? The various therapies, for us, were disappointingly ineffectual. I had observed firsthand her improvement when we removed gluten and casein from her diet, and so I decided to find out whether she was reacting to any other foods or environmental factors. In early April, I decided to get more bloodwork done. Probing by the doctor and needle pricks were not easy for Taylor. Each blood draw required an entire day of prepping, calming, and then rewarding her once we were through with the ordeal. And on more than one occasion I loitered in the medical center's parking lot, dealing with an uncontrollable child melting down from the unacceptable insult of a syringe needle. I remember wrestling Taylor into her car seat in the back, naively thinking all was contained, though not quiet. Then she began to bang her toy against the window while screaming. I had to stop the car, not even making it out of the parking lot. I pulled into another parking spot and moved her car seat to the middle so she couldn't reach the windows. Nothing would calm her down. I felt like I was in a horror movie, and I'm sure anyone who witnessed the scene was horrified, too.

The lab results were helpful in that we discovered that Taylor was allergic to cats, dogs, and dust mites. Banning our beloved kitty from the bedrooms did not help with any of Taylor's behaviors, but it did appear to provide some relief from her nighttime sniffles. Her IgE and IgG (immunoglobulin) antibody levels were elevated, suggesting a high level of inflammation. However, the tests indicated that she did not have any allergies or sensitivities to foods, including wheat and milk. This was surprising to me, considering how Taylor's behavior had improved on the GF/CF diet. Yet, despite not testing positive for these antigens, clearly Taylor benefited by removing gluten and casein from her diet. The protein chemist in me wondered: What was going on in her body with these proteins? What would cause behavior changes when there was no antibody response?

Around the time of the blood testing, my mom and I started to notice that Taylor would occasionally stop what she was doing and stare blankly into space for short periods. I'd wave my hands in front of her eyes and get no reaction. The episodes would last only 5 to 15 seconds. Kids do "zone out" sometimes, but Taylor's episodes would happen mid-sentence or, frighteningly, mid-step up a ladder on a play structure. I discussed this "spacing out" with a close friend who occasionally suffered from a type of epilepsy called *absence seizures*, which is characterized by a brief loss of consciousness. The person experiencing an absence seizure is often unaware of it, and I wondered if that was what was happening here. Mitch was dismissive and didn't observe the behavior or have the same interpretation. Still, together we decided to take Taylor to a neurologist, hoping to get an explanation for these strange episodes and maybe even the yes/no loops, which had always struck me as seizure-like because it seemed she was "stuck" in a loop.

We were fortunate to have access to Stanford's Lucile Packard Children's Hospital, a facility known for its outstanding neurology unit. We consulted with a neurologist who recommended Taylor get an electroencephalogram (EEG). An EEG records the brain's electrical activity, which can be evaluated for abnormal activity. For an EEG to detect absence seizures, a seizure must occur during the test. The test itself was a sad experience, involving 50 electrodes attached all over Taylor's head. Taylor was not a happy camper.

During the procedure, an EEG technician collected brainwave patterns while Taylor was subjected to a strobe light, shown different visual patterns, and allowed to rest and read books. One week later, Mitch, Taylor, and I returned to Stanford to review the results of her EEG test. A group of interns attended the appointment along with the lead doctor.

The neurologist reported that no seizure activity had been detected during the EEG, nor was there any evidence of past grand mal epileptic seizures. The neurologist also stated that she had observed slow wave patterns in the EEG recording of Taylor's brain, an observation consistent with developmental delays. The neurologist provided no further explanation for this finding, and I remember thinking that I needed to research brain frequencies and learn about "slow wave patterns." Great, another piece of the puzzle to sort out.

One month after Taylor's EEG test, we received the official neurology report from Stanford. The report repeated the neurologist's observation of "slow wave patterns consistent with developmental delays" and added that "diffuse slowing is a nonspecific finding and classically indicates encephalopathy." I found the reference to encephalopathy intriguing and added that to my list of things to learn about.

Encephalopathy, I learned, is a general term for a disorder of the brain stemming from various causes, which could be genetic, autoimmune, brain trauma, infection, or a metabolic disorder. "Diffuse slow wave patterns" was associated with brain inflammation. The question in Taylor's case was "what was the cause of the slow brain waves, and was it reversible?" I decided, therefore, to focus my reading on brain inflammation and ways to reduce it.

I quickly learned that brain inflammation adversely impacts brain function in numerous ways. It is the underlying pathology in illnesses as varied as mood disorders, inability to focus, migraines, hyperactivity, autism, Alzheimer's disease . . . the list goes on. I wondered: Could the improvements we had observed so far with the GF/CF diet reflect a reduction in brain inflammation? Could there be, perhaps, something beyond gluten, casein, and nutritional deficiencies that was inflaming her brain?

I knew an inflamed brain is not optimal for learning, and my new mantra became "fix the brain, then retrain."

May 2010

I had my quest: find the connection between diet and inflammation of the brain. I began by searching for scientific articles specifically on autism and diet, but other than the GF/CF diet, there was (and remains) very little scientific research in this area. I found myself going back to reading blogs. One blog discussing autism and GF/CF diets—and I don't even recall the author or website—contained comments made by parents of autistic children, sharing their experience of what was working and what wasn't. As I'd found before, parents' experiences with the GF/CF diet seemed to be inconsistent, but a fair number of them reported some improvement in their autistic child's behaviors with diet. Then I read a comment that would change the course of my family's life.

One parent wrote that his autistic son benefited from removing not only gluten and casein from his diet but also monosodium glutamate (MSG). My initial response was "who the heck would feed their kid, especially one with special needs, MSG?" My epiphany didn't occur right away, but the seed was planted on that late evening while I mentally dismissed this dad's observation.

The next morning, I was rummaging through the refrigerator deciding what to feed Taylor for breakfast. I pulled out some organic chicken apple sausages. Something struck me about the previous night's reading and the MSG comment, and I decided to review the ingredients: "Organic Chicken, Organic Dried Apples, Sodium Lactate (from Beets). Contains Less Than 2% of the following: Sea Salt, Organic Apple Juice Concentrate, Organic Spices, Organic Garlic."

Realizing that I didn't understand all the ingredients listed on the package, I decided to use Google Scholar to search for scientific articles on autism and glutamate (glutamate is the same thing as monosodium glutamate, MSG). While Taylor's now suspect organic chicken sausage sizzled in the fry pan, I began the investigation that brought me to the epiphany that has come to define my life's mission. The scientific literature was abundantly clear: from the gut to the brain, excess glutamate signaling ("signaling" is when glutamate in the body causes nerve cells to fire) has been implicated in many neurological and inflammatory disorders. But as I was to learn later that morning, and many other mornings and days spent researching the scientific literature in the months and years to come, excess glutamate signaling wasn't just limited to autism. Excess glutamate signaling is implicated in many diseases, such as multiple sclerosis, depression, Parkinson's, Alzheimer's, and rheumatoid arthritis. And so much more. Excess glutamate signaling is such a pervasive hallmark of disease that I was struck by the sheer number of basic research and clinical studies that attempt to prevent or treat various diseases with drugs that block (prevent) glutamate from binding to its target cells.

At this point, I was doing a deep research dive. As a scientist, I wanted to understand exactly what glutamate did in the body, in health and disease; as a mother I wanted to quickly understand how this related to the food I was feeding my family.

For the first time, I decided to question every single ingredient in Taylor's entire diet. Could any of these be sources of glutamate? In the package of organic sausages, what was "sodium lactate from beets"? How was the sodium lactate produced? Was the chicken processed in some way? Using Google Patents, I started investigating manufacturing patents for common ingredients in our foods that I had never questioned. Even though I thought our diet was healthy, I came to realize that I didn't truly understand what I was feeding Taylor—or our entire family for that matter—because food labels are vague. Clearly, my journey needed to go beyond science, and I embarked on a full-fledged investigation of the food industry. What I discovered was deeply unsettling. But I am getting ahead of my story. To understand the significance of what I was learning, I had to know how glutamate affects the body.

What I learned is that one of glutamate's many critical roles in the body is that of *neurotransmitter*. This means glutamate is naturally released from our own human cells to send messages to other regions of the body. That's the "signaling" I alluded to earlier. When our nervous system encounters danger, glutamate sends out the signal, and the body launches its defense in the form of inflammation.

What this means is foods that are inflammatory cause glutamate to be released from our own human cells. At this point you may be saying, "Huh?" I'll go into this connection in more detail in chapter 6, "The Slow-Growing Fire: Inflammation and Diet." Suffice it to say, I learned enough early on to give me the idea to try another experiment. I wanted to determine the effects of removing foods that contained free glutamate (MSG), whether or not labeled as such, from our diet.

Late May 2010

I was consumed with planning the experiment over the following weeks. The food lifestyle approach that evolved from this I later called the REID protocol, which stands for Reduced Excitatory Inflammatory Diet. REID is also my last name, so I'm sure not to forget the letters. I will refer to this protocol as such going forward, but of course the word REID wasn't coined at the time I embarked on my experiment.

My experimental design was simple: remove foods that contained free glutamate (MSG) from the diet. The execution, on the other hand, was enormously difficult. Mitch was extremely resistant to this next phase of our dietary journey. We argued and debated quite a bit about the direction in which I was heading. He once again said we needed to seek "real" help for Taylor and stop wasting our time on her food. "Taylor's autism has nothing to do with her diet!" he protested, as I carefully examined the list of ingredients in his favorite cereal and excluded it from Taylor's new diet.

I knew at the time that Mitch viewed my efforts as a personal attack on him and a rejection of the familiar foods that provided him comfort. He argued that my views were not fair to Taylor. I argued the virtues of just letting me try this approach. After some exhausting debates, I promised Mitch that if we didn't see improvement in Taylor over a one-month period, I would do as he wished and call the behavioral therapist recommended by the Stanford medical team. I had one month and one shot to execute my experiment.

The clock was ticking. I proceeded to remove almost every single packaged food product from our pantry and refrigerator. All sauces, condiments, dressings, soups, and broths were squirreled away. Sometimes I would resort to investigating an unknown ingredient using Google Patents or looking up manufacturing processes for ingredients. If the ingredient was suspect, it was removed. I set up a shelf in the pantry and one in the refrigerator labeled "Taylor's Food." That this was a major overhaul in our diet is an understatement, if there ever was one! I thought removing gluten and casein was a major dietary change, but this way of approaching food was on a whole new level. I had to redefine my *definition* of food. As I didn't want Taylor to go through this experiment alone, I, too, planned on eating the same foods.

The results were dramatic and immediate. From the point I implemented REID, Taylor never again had one of her yes/no loops. In contrast, in the week before we started REID—right in the middle of one of my and Mitch's debates—Taylor had one of the worst yes/no loop episodes that I can remember. That was the last one. Within days of starting what would become our new food lifestyle, her anxiety started to subside and she appeared calmer and "comfortable in her skin." It is incredibly difficult to describe how it was as if a cloud had lifted and she was seeing the world differently—her new awareness was so apparent in her eyes and facial expressions. Taylor was now attentive when her name was spoken, became interested in people's conversations, and developed newfound interest in her surroundings. I knew we were on the right track.

This new food lifestyle was hard. During the first week of the diet, I was increasingly irritable as I felt food withdrawals. I craved many of my favorite processed foods, especially brie and bread, and I found myself circling the kitchen wondering what to eat. Taylor was visibly frustrated that she wasn't being served foods she requested or craved. I found myself telling my almost-four-year-old that the store had stopped selling her favorite foods.

The effort was all worth it. Over the next few weeks, a new little girl emerged, one increasingly curious and ready to explore her world. All the rituals that made it so challenging to get through the day either disappeared or were easily managed. Taylor started eating foods that she'd previously refused to eat, accepting a variety of foods and textures. Nut butters could now have chunks of nuts in them. Broccoli was consumed without protest. After years of accommodation and conflict, this was nothing short of shocking.

June 2010

At this point, Taylor was two months shy of her fourth birthday. Taylor's language skills exploded as spontaneous conversation filled the room. At her special needs school, one of Taylor's Individual Education Plan (IEP) goals was for her to start using multi-word sentences. Three weeks into her new diet, she was using complex sentences, communicating her needs, and asking questions and understanding responses. This rapid development, her speech therapist noted, was highly unusual.

The best way I can describe the first month after we started REID is that it seemed like the learning channels in Taylor's brain suddenly opened, enabling her to better receive information. She began asking questions about her world. "What's that?" was a now frequent refrain. She had never asked a question before this point! She started getting dressed by herself, going to the bathroom without assistance, and washing her hands and face without constant supervision and prodding. At the one month "check-in" with my husband, we agreed the food lifestyle changes were benefiting Taylor's overall health and significantly improving symptoms associated with autism. Not that I still didn't face many challenges in partnering with my husband to comply with the REID food lifestyle.

July 2010

The second month into REID, I focused even more intently on identifying MSG (free glutamate) in food products, supplements, medicines, and body products (yes, body products such as lotions, and even oral care products such as toothpaste). I either found replacements, made my own, or did without. Taylor's use and comprehension of language continued to expand dramatically. Her sound and visual sensitivities subsided and eventually ceased altogether.

As another benefit, Taylor's allergies to cats and dust were significantly reduced. Taylor could now touch the cat and even snuggle with our furry family member without consequence.

I also experienced significant health benefits. My transition to a REID lifestyle, however, was at first less than pleasant. I had headaches for about three days, coinciding with my strongest cravings for foods containing MSG (i.e., most processed foods). Even after eating, I often felt hungry. I stayed with it, though, and every time I craved processed food I would reach for raw nuts or carrots instead. After those initial few days, I started to notice improvements. My low-level headaches, which I had lived with all my life, ceased. Pollen allergies that had required allergy shots when I was younger completely disappeared. I shed weight, had more energy, and no longer experienced the "brain fogs" and "food comas" I now recognize as being associated with eating specific foods. My disposition changed, becoming more positive, optimistic, and energetic. Paradoxically, I was entering a phase of my life where I was committing myself to spending even more time on food preparation and cooking, but this huge time commitment did not distress me. My complicated life suddenly seemed easier to manage.

Taylor had started at her special needs school at the end of February, and we began REID in May. By the end of the school year in early June, Taylor's teachers recommended she attend a mainstream preschool. One therapist said that "Taylor would be bored if she continued at the special needs school." At first, Mitch and I were concerned that Taylor's improvements might not be sustainable. Having worked so hard to get special needs services, we didn't want to give up Taylor's spot in the special needs school, only to find out later she still needed the services. Happily, this was not the case. As we would learn, her new behaviors were sustainable, if we adhered to our new dietary lifestyle.

Today

Back in 2010, when we began our food journey, I desperately hoped that my instincts and scientific training would lead me to a way to help my child. Today I am an unabashed convert to the notion that food is our solution. As I spoke to others—both in person and online—something very interesting happened. I learned that our story was not unique. Many people had found that eating the "wrong" food caused their health issues, and that an overhaul in diet was the basis of their healing. The stories were many and varied, but there was a consistent theme: *what one ate mattered*. In many cases, the impact of food on one's quality of life was profound. It became my mission to raise awareness of this issue, and to do that I founded my nonprofit, Unblind My Mind.

In this book, I've tried my best to assemble and explain the evidence that connects dietary glutamate to disease in a way that you don't have be an expert to understand. In chapter 1, we look at the statistics that describe the state of health in the United States and examine what science says about the role of processed foods in making people sick.

In chapters 2 and 3, I introduce you to glutamate and explain how it's created during food manufacturing and why it is added to so many processed foods. I'll show you the numbers, and you'll see just how much MSG you are ingesting, unaware. And I will introduce you to the players in the glutamate industry who want to keep things exactly the way they are, where concerns about MSG are stifled, labels aren't transparent, and consumers believe that the level of glutamate in the food they eat is natural and safe.

In chapters 4 through 7, we get into biology. In these chapters you will learn that glutamate functions as a neurotransmitter in the body, and too much glutamate is toxic to cells. I will explain why glutamate dysregulation is associated with so many modern ailments—obesity, depression, diabetes, chronic inflammation, and autism, among them—and tie this to the very important role your gut microbiome plays in health and disease. I'll also share with you case studies of people suffering from some of these conditions who have been helped through REID food recommendations.

Finally, in chapter 8 I will show you how you can take control of your diet and change your life for the better. I'll be your guide, providing you with a roadmap and outlining steps and goals—and tips for navigating social situations that will inevitably occur when you don't eat what everyone else is eating.

My journey started with a severe illness, my daughter's autism. I now realize how making the wrong food choices can be devasting to health, and how that can affect a family. Your situation may be similar or different, but whatever it is, I know it is deeply personal. I hope the information in these pages provides insight and guidance wherever you are on your journey. What I learned did not fix everything in my life, however. If you are wondering if the dramatic improvement in my daughter's autism symptoms was all that was needed for Mitch and me to have a stress-free, happy marriage, well, it was not. I am grateful to Mitch for eventually coming around to my perspective, to the point of defending Taylor's glutamate-free diet to all challengers, but he and I are now divorced. I share this detail in the same spirit of transparency that I share the story about my family throughout this book.

I

The Crisis Is Real

You don't have to read very far to see that I have painted a bull's-eye on processed and ultraprocessed food. We now have scientific evidence that processed food is bad for you, but exactly how is it making us sick, and what can we do about it? This book makes the case that processed food compromises health not just because of added sugar, salt, and fat, but also because of its load of added glutamate. Glutamate gives food the taste sensation known as *umami*. Glutamate has many names: monosodium glutamate, MSG, glutamic acid, but it also appears in food labels as hydrolyzed yeast extract, hydrolyzed protein, spices, and is even included in ingredients as healthy sounding as natural flavors. The reason why glutamate is in so many products is because, in our bodies, glutamate works as an *excitatory neurotransmitter*—we'll get into the science of that later—but functionally, this means that glutamate sends a pleasure signal to the brain.[1] Unfortunately, when glutamate is used as a food additive, it makes foods addictive. Think about junk food, which has little nutritional value but is manufactured to be nearly irresistible.

The molecule glutamate itself is not a bad actor. It is everywhere in the body and plays a critical role in learning, balancing the metabolic needs of cells, and triggering a healthy immune response. The problem arises when there is too much glutamate in our bodies and glutamate becomes *dysregulated* (another technical word that will be explained later in this book). An out-of-whack glutamate regulatory system lies at the heart of many diseases. Obesity, diabetes, chronic inflammation, autism, addiction, cancer, and the behavioral and cognitive issues crippling modern society can all be characterized as the consequences of a disrupted glutamate regulatory system.

I learned this when my daughter Taylor was diagnosed with autism at the age of three.

When I give presentations describing my experience before an audience, I often start with a very sad video of my little girl having a complete meltdown. In the video Taylor is sobbing, caught in what the family called the dreaded yes/no loop. It's a state of cognitive confusion, when a child simultaneously wants something to happen and not to happen. The first episode of the yes/no loop occurred when my older daughter was helping Taylor wash up before bedtime. Taylor started what appeared to be a game, insisting that her sister turn the water on and then turn the water off. Unfortunately, neither water on nor water off seemed to be the right choice, and with each turn of the faucet Taylor became more agitated and distraught. My older daughter tried to end the "game" and said it was time to go to bed. Taylor became hysterical and refused to leave the sink, screaming "on!" and then "off!" despite neither action calming her down. It was a horrible and frightening experience for everyone. In the video I show a similar episode (episodes that were all too frequent in Taylor's young life). You can see the sheer misery in Taylor's face and tiny body. These episodes would last for hours, until she would exhaust herself and fall asleep. Bizarrely, sometimes she would wake up in the middle of the night and resume the yes/no loop behavior while in bed, right where she left off. I now recognize this otherwise inexplicable behavior as the consequence of inflammation in my daughter's brain, which had hijacked her ability to make sense of the world.

When my daughter was diagnosed with autism, moderate on the spectrum, my only goal in life was to find out what I could do to help my child. I am a biochemist, so my first impulse was to study the scientific literature. I discovered that not a lot was known about the causes of autism, nor were there one-size-fits-all success stories recommending therapies and treatments. The saying "once you know a person with autism, you know one person with autism" seemed to apply here. Individuals with autism are just that—individuals. While there is a core set of behaviors that define autism, the response of these behaviors to treatment differs widely.

I did find useful information on online parents' forums. Some parents reported autism symptoms improved with the removal of wheat and dairy from their children's diet. This was referred to as the gluten-free/casein-free (GF/CF) diet, after the main proteins in wheat and dairy. I tried that, and Taylor showed impressive improvements. I detail this in the introduction to this book, but the upshot is that I later discovered that, by removing gluten and casein from my daughter's diet, I was also in effect removing significant sources of glutamate. I vowed to remove all sources of glutamate from our diet to see if that would help manage Taylor's symptoms.

What I then came to realize, after a deep dive into food manufacturing patents and Food and Drug Administration (FDA) regulations, is that we are ingesting far greater amounts of glutamate than you might think, if your guess was based on ingredient labels. As I will show, the vast bulk of dietary glutamate is created during commercial processing of proteins, and because technically it is not something added, it doesn't need to be stated on ingredient labels. Add to that the glutamate that *is* being added to food as an ingredient during the manufacturing process, and the numbers become truly sobering. In 1973, world production of MSG was 13,000 metric tons. In 2022, it was a staggering 3.5 *million* metric tons.[2] Glutamate is entering the food supply, in soups and sauces and juice boxes and soft drinks. What ultimately reversed my daughter's autism diagnosis, and improved the health of our entire family, was eliminating glutamate in processed foods from our diets and replacing it with whole foods.

At the beginning of my presentation, I ask people in the audience for a show of hands: how many consume MSG in their diet? Few, if any, raise their hands. At the end of my presentation, most do.

Since I first discovered the key role glutamate played in inflammation and in provoking my daughter's autism symptoms, I have learned that the health effects of glutamate go way beyond its impact on childhood conditions such as autism, ADHD, developmental delays, and the increasing incidence of mood disorders such as anxiety and depression in pediatric populations. Monosodium glutamate, specifically in processed and ultraprocessed food, is contributing to a health crisis in America that affects everyone, regardless of age.

That America is sick and getting sicker is borne out by the statistics:

- More than two in three adults (73.6 percent) are considered overweight or obese, and 22 percent of kids between the ages of 12 and 19 years are obese.[3]
- More than 13 percent of the U.S. population of all ages has diabetes, and 35 percent have prediabetes. For those 65 and older, 27 percent have diabetes and more than 47 percent are prediabetic.[4]
- More than three-quarters (78 percent) of adults over 55 years old are living with at least one chronic disease such as heart disease, stroke, cancer, or diabetes.[5]
- In any given year, an estimated 26 percent of Americans ages 18 and older suffer from a diagnosable mental disorder. Mental disorders are the leading cause of disabilities worldwide.[6]
- About one in six (17 percent) children ages 3 to 17 years are diagnosed with a developmental disability.[7]
- Over 40 million Americans ages 12 and older suffer from a substance abuse disorder.[8]

Why are we in crisis, sick with so many different illnesses that on the surface seem unrelated? In my experience, the one thing the vast majority of chronic diseases have in common is that their pathologies manifest as inflammation. This is true of Alzheimer's disease, depression, autism, addiction, heart disease, diabetes, cancer, pain—even obesity has an inflammatory component. The reason I am painting a target on processed and ultraprocessed food is that these foods, with their high complement of glutamate, are pro-inflammatory. That makes them a serious threat to health.

The results from multiple peer-reviewed scientific studies[9] that have followed hundreds of thousands of participants over decades make the health risks of ultraprocessed food abundantly clear. Consumption of ultraprocessed food significantly increases the risk of obesity and death by cardiovascular disease, cancer, and stroke.[10]

Consuming ultraprocessed food increased the risk of death by *all* causes—by as much as 62 percent.[11]

With the health risks of ultraprocessed food so clear, should we worry about how these foods are impacting our youth, whose developing brains and bodies are particularly sensitive to the excitotoxic effects of glutamate? The data shout YES. A 2021 report published in the prestigious *Journal of the American Medical Association* studying almost 34,000 U.S. youths from 2 to 19 years old found that two-thirds—67 percent—of total calories consumed was from ultraprocessed food. This is concerning, when juxtaposed with what we know about the burgeoning incidences of developmental delays, behavioral issues, diabetes, and obesity in pediatric populations.

The solution seems simple enough. For individuals, this means eliminating processed food from the diet and replacing it with whole foods—preferably organic, and predominantly plant-based. As a nation, this means setting dietary standards for processed food and requiring the glutamate content be fully disclosed on food labels. Why is this so hard to do?

And that is the crux of it.

In the same way Big Tobacco obfuscated the health risks of smoking, and the fossil fuel industry injected doubt into the science of human-caused climate change, the processed food industry has engaged in a well-funded campaign to discredit the scientific evidence that MSG poses a risk. Big Food would have you believe the science is settled. It is not. My reason for writing this book is to present the science and the evidence to empower you, the reader, to choose how to optimize your health.

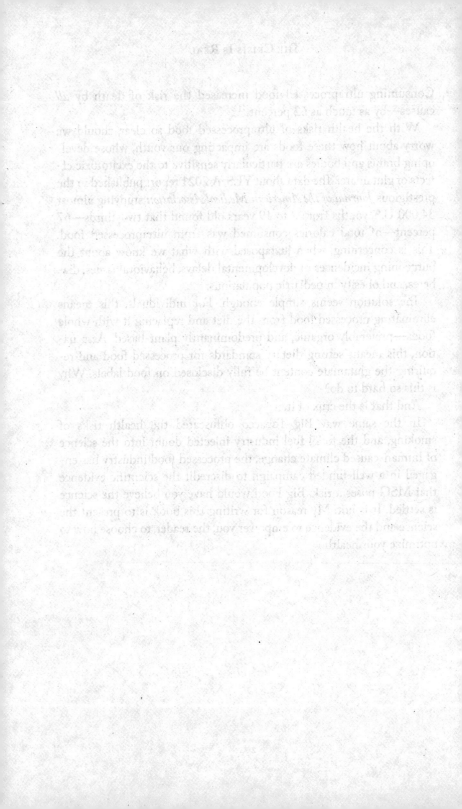

2

Can't Eat Just One

WHEN I REMOVED GLUTEN AND CASEIN PROTEINS FROM TAYLOR'S diet, she improved, but even with the improvement she would have been diagnosed with autism. She still exhibited the extremely dysfunctional behaviors such as the yes/no loop where, once she got into an obsessive indecision loop, she couldn't exit it without exhausting herself from screaming and negative emotions. Her slight improvements in health, though, were enough to turn me into a detective, and it kept me researching and questioning the effect of other proteins in her diet.

And we had plenty of other proteins in the diet. I wondered why so many people benefited from the removal of gluten and casein from the diet (Taylor and myself included), but many others did *not* feel better. In my search for answers, I recalled the blog I had stumbled across earlier, discussing GF/CF diets for those with autism, where a father reported that his child with autism benefited not only from removal of gluten and casein, but also monosodium glutamate. While my first reaction was that we had no MSG in our diet, and this comment didn't apply to our family, the seed was planted in my mind to find out just exactly what *was* in our diet. I started to question all of the various ingredients in factory-processed food and realized that I really had no idea what "beet extract" in our sausage was or how the meat was processed, or what gluten-free natural flavor in our seemingly healthy cookie treat was. After examining many food patents

29

and researching gluten and casein proteins, I identified one very significant variable, which can explain why some people benefit from removing gluten and casein, and others don't. In home kitchens, as well as in clinical trials, what hasn't been measured when examining the benefit of GF/CF diets is the amount of free glutamate that still remains in the diet, even after removal of gluten and casein proteins. And as I learned, that can be a lot. Manufacturing processes that increase the availability of free glutamate from *all* proteins in food (not just gluten and casein proteins), as well as patented recipes that add glutamate directly to food, have become essential to making food appealing and marketable.

This chapter and the next describe what I call America's glutamate problem. At issue is the reformulation of food that has occurred over the last few decades, and the food industry practices that have resulted in the glutamation of our nation. A look at the numbers—the amount of MSG in modern diets—and the players—those with a vested interest in MSG—give you a very different narrative from what is being broadcasted. I hope these two chapters will give you what you need to know to outmaneuver Big Food, despite the money and effort being spent to keep the consumer blinded.

Glutamate Goes by Different Names

There are a few basics to get straight before we delve deeper into glutamate and food. Understand these and you will see through a common misconception perpetuated by the food industry, which would have you believe that the MSG in a bottle labeled "MSG" bears no relation to the free glutamate that food manufacturers liberally add to food or the MSG generated from proteins during processing. In fact, they are functionally the same in the body.

Glutamate is an amino acid, one of 20 common amino acids that are the building blocks of proteins. Glutamate exists either by itself as "free glutamate," or it can be chemically bonded with other amino acids in proteins. Depending on the environment (i.e., if glutamate is dissolved in water, or if it is in a solid form, or if the pH is high or low), glutamate has a variety of names, as shown in figure 2.1.

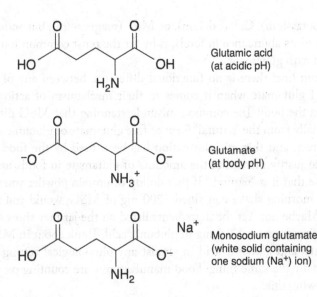

Glutamic acid
(at acidic pH)

Glutamate
(at body pH)

Monosodium glutamate
(white solid containing
one sodium (Na⁺) ion)

Figure 2.1 Glutamic acid, glutamate, and monosodium glutamate (MSG) are different names for the same substance.

The top structure in figure 2.1 is glutamic acid, and the middle structure is glutamate. The bottom structure is called monosodium glutamate (MSG) because it is glutamate with a single ion of sodium (Na^+). (Note that sodium is a component of table salt, which has the chemical name sodium chloride, $NaCl$.) MSG is created when a negatively charged glutamate molecule forms a bond with a positively charged sodium ion (Na^+). MSG is a convenient form of glutamate for sprinkling on your food or for food manufacturers to utilize because it is a white powder—a kind of salt—that dissolves easily in water.

In the body or in food, MSG becomes simply glutamate, because when MSG dissolves, the Na^+ ion leaves the compound. How does that work? Think about how salt crystals—$NaCl$—dissolve when you add salt to water. In the same way that $NaCl$ dissolves into Na^+ and Cl^- in water (and in your mouth), MSG dissolves into Na^+ and glutamate. Glutamate can also bond with other positively charged ions, such as K^+ (potassium), Ca^{2+} (calcium), or Mg^{2+} (magnesium), but sodium, because of its abundance in foods, is by far the most common ion associated with glutamate.

Bottom line: there is no functional difference between any of the forms of glutamate when it comes to their mechanism of action or effect on the body. The common misunderstanding that MSG differs functionally from the "natural" form of free glutamate or glutamic acid is incorrect, and this misinformation has been used by the food industry to justify increasing the amounts of glutamate in foods under the guise that it is "natural." If that dollop of protein powder you add to your morning shake contained 1200 mg of MSG, would you still use it? Maybe not. Yet the ingredients listed on the jar may show that one serving contains 1200 mg of glutamic acid. Think about it: MSG, glutamate, and glutamic acid in almost any physiological setting are functionally the same thing. Food manufacturers are counting on you not knowing this.

I have called out a number of food manufacturers on this false flag, only to be dismissed out of hand. My efforts certainly did not result in more transparency in food ingredient labels. This is important for everyone to understand because excess glutamate in the diet is linked to myriad diseases, obesity being one. I discuss this link in chapter 7, but here's a piece of information that helps connect the dots. A lot of what we've learned about obesity in humans stems from experiments with obese lab rats and mice. How are many of these experimental test subjects created? For over 30 years, it has been a standard laboratory practice to feed lab animals MSG to make them obese,[1] an experiment we seem to be conducting at our own dinner tables today.

MSG Enters the Food Supply

So how did MSG enter the food supply? In 1907, a Japanese professor named Kikunae Ikeda began a research project to identify the substance in kelp that produced a unique taste called *umami* that was favored in soup stocks in Japan. In 1908, he identified the savory umami taste component of kelp as glutamate. In 1909, the monosodium salt of glutamate—MSG—was packaged as a seasoning and given the trademark name Ajinomoto®. This company still exists today and is a major producer of MSG worldwide. Interestingly, the initial process used to manufacture MSG as a food additive used gluten—the wheat protein—because wheat gluten had the highest total glutamate content (>30 grams glutamate/100 grams protein) among industrially available raw materials.[2] In fact, glutamate derives its name from gluten, because this amino acid was first discovered in wheat gluten in 1866 by the German chemist Karl Heinrich Ritthausen. (Truly, as I learned this, it seemed as if everything I needed to connect the dots was hiding in plain sight, discoverable with the simplest online search.)

MSG entered the U.S. market in force in the 1930s. From the mid-1930s until the start of World War II, the United States bought more Ajinomoto flavoring (MSG) than any other country outside of Japan and Taiwan. Demand for MSG came not from individual consumers but rather from companies that made factory-processed foods. Demand for MSG also came from food service industries that supported the U.S. military, which recognized the capacity of MSG to make bland, inexpensive foods flavorful.[3]

Figure 2.2 is telling. In 1970, annual world production of MSG was just over 13,000 metric tons. Today, the annual world production of MSG is estimated to be more than 3.5 *million* metric tons! People, of course, are consuming this staggering amount of MSG, and it represents a fundamental change in the modern diet not seen before 1975. To put this in perspective, enough MSG is manufactured per year to feed every person on earth (8 billion and counting) an estimated 1.2 g of MSG per day.

When safety concerns regarding MSG were made public in the late 1960s, MSG in the food supply went into stealth mode. Food manufacturers weren't willing to remove this ingredient. Why? It's their secret ingredient that turns otherwise tasteless food into something that is addictive. And "addictive" is exactly the correct word here. As described in chapter 3, "Safety Concerns and Business Interests Collide," political and financial interests have long worked together to ensure this ingredient remains in the food supply. Corporations exert extraordinary influence over food regulatory bodies and control how glutamate is labeled, or not labeled.

33

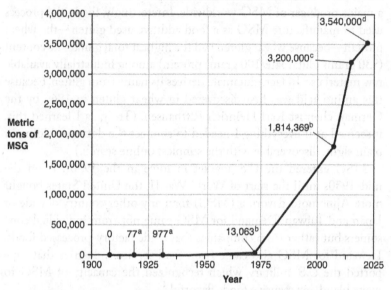

Annual Global Production of MSG

[a]Sand, Jordan. "A Short History of MSG: Good Science, Bad Science, and Taste Cultures." *Gastronomica* 5, no. 4 (November 2005): 38–49. doi:10.1525/gfc.2005.5.4.38.

[b]Sano, Chiaki. "History of Glutamate Production." *The American Journal of Clinical Nutrition* 90, no. 3 (July 29, 2009): 728S732S. doi:10.3945/ajcn.2009.27462f.

[c]S&P Global. "Global Demand for Flavor Enhancer MSG Grows as Incomes Expand, Cultures Shift, IHS Says," 2014. https://www.spglobal.com/commodityinsights/en/ci/products/-monosodium-glutamate-chemical-economics-handbook.html.

[d]"Global Monosodium Glutamate Production and Consumption from 2021-2022." Maia Research CO, 2022.

Figure 2.2 MSG enters the food supply.

The sobering truth is that the situation is much worse than 3.5 million metric tons of pure MSG in the food supply. The actual amount of MSG in the diet is even greater because MSG comes from many sources other than the food additive labeled "MSG." In fact, pure MSG makes up only a small fraction of the total glutamate consumed by people in modern industrialized nations. The rest of it comes from the way processed foods are manufactured. Put simply, the health issues that arise from excess glutamate consumption in modern diets are a consequence of the numerous sources of free glutamate found in factory-processed foods.

Why are food manufacturers so liberal in their use of glutamate, and defensive of its place in their recipes and our diet? The simple reason is that it makes food taste better, and in the right amounts, makes people eat more. Glutamate's mode of action in the body supports food cravings. In fact, as we will see in chapter 4, the physiological action of glutamate in the body is to make food addicting. And as food manufacturers know, when food is made irresistible, people want more of it, and profits are made.

Proteins, Glutamate, and Processed Food

To become a savvy food consumer, we need to review some basics about protein chemistry. Remember these four points, and everything else makes sense.

1. Proteins are strings of amino acids linked together by peptide bonds. One way to visualize this is by imagining amino acids strung together in a protein chain like beads on a string.
2. Peptide bonds can be broken through a chemical process known as hydrolysis.
3. Hydrolysis occurs in the presence of water, and is facilitated by the addition of acid, base, enzymes, or physical conditions like heat and pressure.
4. The products of protein hydrolysis are free amino acids.

In unprocessed whole foods, most proteins are intact (that is, peptide bonds tie together the amino acids). However, in factory-processed foods, proteins are subjected to processes and conditions that degrade the protein and hydrolyze the peptide bonds. The harsher the processing conditions, the greater the degree to which the peptide bonds are hydrolyzed. The result of industrial processing of proteins in food is free amino acids and short peptides (short strings of amino acids). This is how free glutamate is produced during food manufacturing (figure 2.3).

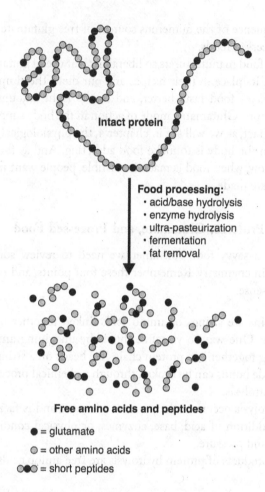

Intact protein

Food processing:
- acid/base hydrolysis
- enzyme hydrolysis
- ultra-pasteurization
- fermentation
- fat removal

Free amino acids and peptides

● = glutamate
○ = other amino acids
○●○ = short peptides

Figure 2.3 Beads on a string. Food processing breaks up the protein strand into free amino acids and short peptides.

To get a feel for whether the food you are eating contains free glutamate, let's start by looking at the food label. Many factory-processed foods have one or more ingredients that contain hydrolyzed proteins (e.g., hydrolyzed vegetable protein, hydrolyzed soy protein, or hydrolyzed yeast extract). Proteins can be hydrolyzed in several ways: by the application of strong acid (e.g., hydrochloric acid) and high heat (e.g., >110°C) for a period of time (e.g., 24 hours), through fermentation, or by the addition of protein enzymes (e.g., papain, endopeptidase, or trypsin). The hydrolysis reaction can break all the protein's peptide bonds, resulting in 100 percent free amino acids. Or, as figure 2.3 shows, the hydrolysis reaction can be partial, resulting in a mixture of free amino acids and short peptides. Assume that if your food label lists hydrolyzed *anything*, your processed food almost certainly contains free glutamate, or at best, short peptides containing glutamate.

Being part of a small peptide doesn't protect glutamate from hydrolysis for very long, however. Once food enters the stomach, short peptides (but not the large proteins that you would get from unprocessed whole foods) are quickly converted to free amino acids—and free glutamate—by stomach acid and the stomach enzyme, pepsin.

Here is an important distinction: when we consume whole fresh foods (foods that have not been factory processed), most of the glutamate we are consuming is "bound glutamate," which is glutamate that is still part of an intact protein. This is how humans ingested most glutamate before food was made in a factory, and as we shall see, this makes an enormous difference to our health.

A Glutamate Primer: Food Processing

So, what are some other processing techniques used by food manufacturers to enrich their products with free glutamate? Let me describe these, using gluten as an example.

Gluten is a class of protein found in wheat, barley, rye, and malts, as well as in triticale and other primitive grains, including kamut and spelt. This protein is an ingredient in a wide variety of foods in the Western diet. Gluten, when isolated from these grains, is used as a food additive in the form of flavoring and can be added to foods as a stabilizing or thickening agent.

Gluten is so named because of its glue-like properties, providing elasticity in breads and baked goods. Compared to wheat varieties that existed not that long ago, modern wheat has extra gluten genes, added through crossbreeding genetics that started in the 1900s. The goal was to provide ever-greater elasticity and protein content to wheat. Today, gluten is also added directly to many wheat products. Breads, for example, are often gluten-fortified to enhance the texture and flavor of the dough. Food manufacturers enrich wheat products with processed gluten to increase their soft, chewy texture. The greater the "doughiness" of a pasta or bread, the more processed gluten has been added to it.

Approximately 30 percent of gluten protein is comprised of glutamate (aka glutamic acid) as part of its protein structure. (Remember, glutamate and glutamic acid are the same amino acid, but when it is part of a protein, glutamate takes the form of glutamic acid, so that is how we'll refer to it now.) Although glutamic acid is one of the most common naturally occurring amino acids in proteins, this abundance is amplified in gluten—30 percent is an extraordinarily high percentage for a single amino acid, when there are 20 amino acids to choose from. Now, if gluten were unprocessed and the protein molecule remained intact, similar to the unbroken "beads on a string" illustrated in figure 2.3, then the glutamic acid would be bound and remain part of the protein. However, we don't consume gluten in a raw, natural, unprocessed form. It gets made into bread, or pasta, and depending on how the food is processed, we end up with different degrees of degraded and hydrolyzed protein. For example, when we bake bread at home, the dough is physically kneaded, fermented with yeast, and baked in the oven, each step breaking down the gluten a little more. During industrial bread production, manufacturing processes degrade the gluten further. The end result is free glutamate in foods that contain gluten.

Here it might be worth examining food manufacturers' use of the phrase "naturally occurring" to describe free glutamate produced during processing. This is a phrase that often shows up in labeling and can be misleading. "Free" is not the natural state of glutamate found in proteins—glutamate (in the form of glutamic acid) is bound to protein by a peptide bond. Food manufacturing processes deliberately degrade gluten and other proteins to free the bound glutamic acid and create MSG. This is one of the secrets of the food industry. Remember the original method used by Ajinomoto in 1909 to manufacture MSG? Ikeda started with wheat gluten, and hydrolyzed it using acid. That process produced MSG.

Today, fermentation is the preferred process for degrading various cheap protein sources and producing free glutamate. Fermentation processes are relatively inexpensive, and carefully selected and genetically engineered yeast and bacteria strains are widely available for industrial-scale use. The microbes used in industrial bread fermentation, for example, are chosen for their ability to release enzymes, which in turn break down the proteins to enrich the glutamic acid/glutamate content in our wheat-based food products (actually, all protein-rich foods). Perhaps most revealing of the goals of food manufacturers, some of these microorganisms are themselves miniature glutamate factories, with the ability to secrete glutamic acid as a byproduct of their metabolism.[4]

What about casein? Casein is a class of proteins found in dairy. Like gluten, casein is rarely consumed raw and contains high levels of glutamic acid—approximately 21 percent of its protein is comprised of glutamate. This is huge compared to the average amount of glutamic acid found in most other proteins, typically between 5 and 10 percent. And like gluten, casein and its many derivatives, such as caseinate, casein hydrolysate, and milk protein extract, are common ingredients in the highly processed foods that typify the Western diet.

What are some common food manufacturing processes that degrade casein proteins? Processes like ultrapasteurization, removal of fats, addition of enzymes, and fermentation result in high levels of free glutamate in many dairy products. To make cheeses, for example, milk is often pasteurized, fermented, and treated with various enzymes to break down the casein proteins and other milk components, giving cheeses their various flavors and aromas. The aging process associated with hard cheeses such as Parmesan also results in degraded milk proteins. Parmigiano Reggiano, because of its long aging and fermentation process, has one of the highest levels of free glutamate among cheeses.

My Aha! moment came when I realized that the issue with the GF/CF diet really didn't have to do with the gluten- and casein-intact proteins, but rather with the free amino acids (primarily glutamate) that are created from these proteins by the food manufacturing process. Specifically, my insight was that broken-down proteins, or hydrolyzed proteins, are a major source of MSG in the diet. In other words, many people can eat the right amount of protein from whole food and not have any ill health effects, but if the protein is already hydrolyzed into smaller pieces, peptides, or individual free amino acids before you take your first bite, then health issues ensue.

The various reported effects of a GF/CF diet therefore contain an important variable that is not accounted for—neither by individuals nor in clinical trials examining the effects of this diet. The variable is *the foods that are replacing the gluten- and casein-containing foods removed from the diet.* If people replaced gluten- and casein-containing foods with other processed foods, which are also sources of free glutamate, then they probably didn't see much benefit because the overall gluta- mate intake isn't reduced enough. However, if the elimination of gluten- and casein-containing foods correlated with increased consumption of whole fresh foods (which contain the low levels of free glutamate with which we evolved), then they probably experienced significant benefit. It wasn't until I understood where all the MSG was coming from that I was able to remove it from our family's diet and experience the health benefits that drastically improved our lives.

The Food Manufacturer's Secret Ingredient

It hasn't been easy to tell the story of how Taylor benefited from what I came to call the Reduced Excitatory Inflammatory Diet (REID) food lifestyle. The science is straightforward, but the trouble arose when I approached food manufacturers with questions about the ingredients in their products. I suppose I was naïve when I started my detective work, as any quick look down the grocery aisle would tell you that the food business is very competitive. Corporations have made huge investments in food products that promote convenience and tastiness over public health, and they did not welcome my inquiries that sug- gested a particular food additive posed a health concern for my family.

In chapter 4, "Overexcited: Glutamate in the Body," I will explain how MSG creates food cravings and why it can be linked to many diseases, including autism. However, the bottom line is that food man- ufacturers put MSG in food because it is addictive. Plain and simple. Adding MSG provides a marketing advantage because it addicts consumers to their product. But disclosing MSG on the label has possible negative marketing consequences for the health-conscious consumer. Ergo, the widespread use of MSG in food is kept secret.

How addictive the food is, and how good our brains think the food tastes, correlates with the amount of free glutamate available to bind to glutamate receptors that reside on our tongues and all throughout our digestive tract. Did you know that the small intestine also has taste receptors, the same type that resides on our tongues? The food industry knows that, and knows how to target them.

MSG is referred to as a flavor enhancer and it imparts to food a flavor often referred to as the fifth taste of umami, but it doesn't have a particular flavor on its own. The higher the MSG content, the more we crave the food. MSG also suppresses satiety—the sense that you are "full," or have had enough to eat. There is a threshold, however, and at some point, adding more MSG decreases food taste.

Entire research and development divisions in food companies have been tasked with finding the "bliss" point where flavor, addiction, and suppressed satiety are optimized in their food products. "Betcha can't eat just one" used to be the tagline for Lay's® brand potato chips commercials. Who knew that the company had fixed that bet by adding addictive ingredients—salt and fat, to be sure, but also MSG—in their best-selling flavored varieties! And the food industry trains our palates at an early age. Despite manufacturers claiming that they removed MSG from infant formula in the 1970s, hydrolyzed proteins and amino acids are still added to formulas. The intent of these additives is to target the glutamate receptors in the small intestine that "increase palatability," or taste preference for the food. By adding these ingredients to infants' first foods, lifetime preferences for MSG-rich foods are formed, and not just for the babies. MSG-rich foods also become the preferred food of the all-important microorganisms in infants' developing gut microbiome, as microflora species become established and gut metabolism adjusts to this glutamate-rich environment.

MSG is just as addictive as sugar and is in just as many foods, yet few are aware of MSG's many names in our foods. Articles such as "The Extraordinary Science of Addictive Junk Food" by Michael Moss[5] reveal just how much research and money goes into making us crave foods. The continued use of MSG by the food industry requires that consumers believe the ingredient safe, and that its presence in food remains covert.

Deception in Food Labels

MSG never recovered from the negative publicity it received in the 1960s. Increased public concern over MSG effectively ended transparency in MSG labeling in food. But while MSG was dropped from labels, the amount of MSG entering our food supply increased, keeping pace with MSG production. Food manufacturers, then and now, are not willing to remove MSG from their products for the simple reason that its addictive properties increase their market share. So manufacturers changed the ways that they added MSG to food.

Before I began my research, I had been under the impression that MSG was mainly added to Chinese restaurant food and, to a limited extent, snack foods. Hence, my initial skepticism to the blog comment about MSG and autism. At that point, I would have flatly denied that anything my family ate contained MSG, especially once we switched to the GF/CF diet. Given the improvements I'd observed in Taylor on the GF/CF diet, I thought that our diet couldn't get much healthier. I was so wrong. The unfortunate fact is that MSG is present in almost all industrially processed foods.

Let's see what the rules say about labeling MSG in food.

The U.S. Food and Drug Administration's (FDA) Code of Federal Regulations is the regulating body for food labels. The FDA requires labeling of all ingredients on processed and packaged foods. Here is a summary of what I found.

The FDA web page specifically dedicated to answering questions about MSG labeling states that when MSG is added to a food, it must be included on the ingredient list as "monosodium glutamate."[6] Glutamate-containing food ingredients, such as hydrolyzed protein and autolyzed yeast extract, also must be listed on food labels. However, when these additives are used, there is no requirement to say on the label that these ingredients contain MSG, only that the manufacturer can no longer say "No MSG" or "No MSG added."

Well, that's *supposed* to be the way manufactures make claims. This sounds like there is some transparency, right? To you, the consumer, I have two messages.

First: Be Aware of Loose Regulations and Enforcement

As mentioned, FDA regulations state that when MSG is added to food, it must be on the list of ingredients. But if you read on, you see this applies only when pure MSG is added as a separate ingredient—as would happen, say, if MSG were poured out of a box and into a vat of broth. The regulations don't require labeling of MSG if it is created during manufacturing.[7] And this is how much of the MSG enters the food supply—during manufacturing, unlabeled, and under the consumer's radar.

To better understand this, I did a deep dive using the search engine Google Patents to investigate a number of the common, vague ingredients listed on labels, such as "natural flavors," "spices," and "hydrolyzed proteins." My sleuthing revealed that loose regulations on ingredient labels can disguise the many ways MSG enters the food supply.

Take "hydrolyzed protein." Remember, if your processed food label lists hydrolyzed *anything,* your food almost certainly contains free glutamate or, at best, short peptides containing glutamate. Short peptides quickly become free amino acids—and free glutamate—in the stomach through the action of stomach acid and the stomach enzyme, pepsin.

I found it eye-opening to learn that as long as an ingredient contains less than 98 percent pure glutamic acid, FDA regulations don't require food manufacturers to list MSG on the label. Food manufacturers are allowed to simply call the ingredient "hydrolyzed soy protein product" or a slew of other names described later in the chapter. These loose labeling standards allow manufacturers to mislead the consumer; because the FDA does not require the amount of total free glutamate to be on the product label, most people have no idea what ingredients or foods contain free glutamate, and at what levels. In fact, the FDA maintains that there is no need for such a requirement because free glutamate is in some natural foods. Yet the amounts of glutamate in many enriched and fortified processed foods are far beyond natural, and by "natural" I mean the amount with which humans evolved.

Now consider "yeast extract." Before I began investigating what's in our food, I never thought to question what "yeast extract" meant. I've learned since that many yeast strains used in food manufacturing are genetically engineered to excrete glutamate, but because this source of free glutamate is "natural" (wrap your head around that one!), food manufacturers are not required to label the product as containing added MSG. In reality, "yeast extract" is a concentrated source of free glutamate, where the contents of glutamate-producing yeast cells are poured into food. Be suspicious of any label containing the word "extract," because it may be an enriched source of glutamate.

Take the fermentation process. As with yeast extract, fermentation of our foods is another source of free glutamate in the diet. In fact, in the United States today, fermentation of corn is how pure MSG (glutamic acid) is produced commercially in food manufacturing facilities and chemical plants. There is no requirement to state whether a food has been fermented on the label. The amount of free glutamate produced this way is dependent on the fermentation time, the microbes used for fermentation, and the amount of protein in the original food. For example—and there are many to choose from—let us examine pork. It took me about two years to figure out why Taylor would have slight reactions to every bacon brand I could find. I searched high and low for just pork and salt as the bacon ingredients, and still, she would have slight reactions. I found the same reaction with ham. But I did not observe reactions to other pork cuts, like pork chops, pork roast, or pork belly. After some further detective work, I determined that the variable causing Taylor to react was whether the meat was cured and/or fermented. Bacon and ham are cured pork, and this process increases the free glutamate content. This is true even for bacon labeled "uncured," as I found out after purchasing uncured bacon and observing the same reaction. When I inquired further with one manufacturer as to their process for uncured bacon, the company stated that they put salt on the pork as a "dry rub" and let it sit at room temperature. I suspect the length of time that the meat sits at room temperature is just under the time that would be required to label the meat "cured." I have yet to understand the difference between this "dry rub" process and curing, but the bacon package states uncured, and still my daughter reacted.

Now take "cultures." What does it mean when the ingredient list includes "cultures"? There are various ways that cultures or microbial strains are labeled on packages, and if they are listed on the label, know that the foods are fermented, and fermentation of protein will create MSG.

What about "spices"? Spice labels disguise another potential source of free glutamate, depending on the spice manufacturing process. The FDA code of regulations has specific requirements for the "spice" or "spices" label. On the face of it, this regulation seems to protect both consumers and manufacturers, since the broad term "spices" allows manufacturers to protect their proprietary blends without revealing trade secrets. Okay, that seems fine. A "spice" label may truly mean something contains just oregano and rosemary. However, use of this catchall term also allows manufacturers to obscure the presence of free glutamate in their products. Not all spice manufacturing processes are created equal, and some ingredients under "spices" may be processed in such a way as to create glutamate. For example, powdered foods like garlic powder or onion powder often contain additional stabilizing, sulfating, enzymatic, and/or anticaking additives—all of which can generate MSG—and these additives can be listed as "spices" on an ingredient label. If you put something like raw garlic through this degradation process, the 12 percent protein in garlic is broken down, freeing amino acids—approximately 24 percent of which is glutamic acid.

I now buy products only when spice ingredients are transparent and listed by their names: oregano, rosemary, turmeric, and so on.

Second: Be Aware of Misleading Claims on Food Products

To recap the food packaging labeling loophole I described earlier, food manufacturers are only required to include the MSG in the list of ingredients if the glutamate added is pure MSG. This has encouraged some manufacturers to make claims that food is free of MSG, even when other ingredients known to contain MSG are present. You frequently see claims of "No MSG Added" or "No MSG" that are questionable, despite FDA regulations against misleading claims.

Some food manufacturers are becoming more transparent, but they are still not 100 percent compliant with FDA rules, in my opinion. For instance, a label for organic chicken broth could state "No MSG Added." Such a label might add a disclaimer such as "A small amount of glutamate naturally occurs in yeast extract." My first thought is, how many people would know that glutamate is the same thing as MSG? The label should plainly state that yeast extract contains MSG. After all, yeast extract is added to foods as a flavor enhancer *because* it contains MSG. My second thought is that products shouldn't be allowed to claim "No MSG added" when a number of common ingredients—and not just yeast extract—contain MSG. For example, if a product contains dehydrated chicken broth or chicken stock, it likely contains free glutamate created during processing. "Natural flavors" is another likely source of free glutamate (more on this later). The point is, we don't know the total free glutamate in the broth because there is no requirement for it to be labeled. At the time of this writing, despite the FDA stating that a manufacturer is not permitted to add "No MSG Added" if ingredients contain MSG, the regulation is not truly enforced. Even the most dedicated label reader could not be faulted for considering our hypothetical chicken broth to be a healthy eating choice, containing negligible amounts of MSG, when in fact it does contain MSG in amounts that are not disclosed.

Moving on to another obfuscation: consider protein powders, protein bars, and protein shakes. In this case, factory processing of the proteins is the source of hidden MSG. When Taylor and I began our smoothie routine, I wanted a protein source and thought of adding protein powders—until I read the patents. Protein powders are growing in popularity in the United States as consumers become obsessed with protein enrichment in the diet. Many protein-powder manufacturers contribute significant amounts of MSG to their customers' diets, and as table 2.1 shows, the proof of that is right on the label.

To our bodies, free glutamic acid is indistinguishable from MSG. The protein powder discussed here delivers more than 3.7 grams of MSG *per serving*. It astonishes me that a food product can contain this amount of MSG and not be required to state explicitly on the

Table 2.1. Amino Acid Profile Per Serving of a Popular Protein Powder

Amino acid	Amount	Amino acid	Amount
Alanine	1150 mg	Lysine	2080 mg
Arginine	568 mg	Methionine	560 mg
Aspartic Acid	2325 mg	Phenylalanine	742 mg
Cysteine	687 mg	Proline	1110 mg
Glutamic Acid	3729 mg	Serine	831 mg
Glutamine	75 mg	Threonine	1238 mg
Glycine	393 mg	Tryptophan	459 mg
Histidine	417 mg	Tyrosine	767 mg
Isoleucine	1332 mg	Valine	1222 mg
Leucine	2597 mg		

Note: According to the numbers provided on the label, reproduced here, a typical serving of this protein powder contains 3,729 mg—that is, 3.729 grams—of glutamic acid. Glutamic acid is the same thing as glutamate, also known as MSG.

label, "Contains MSG." So beware of the contents of protein powders, protein bars, protein chips, protein shakes, or processed protein whatever, as these products likely contain significant amounts of free glutamate.

Another Red Flag Is Enzymes in Food

Enzymes are biological molecules that help break down chemical bonds. If an enzyme capable of breaking the peptide bonds between amino acids in proteins is added to foods that contain protein, significant amounts of free amino acids will be generated, and one of the most abundant amino acids is glutamate. However, "enzymes" listed as an ingredient can indicate any number of different chemical reactions, and without more transparency, we don't know what these enzymes are doing beyond chewing up our food to a predigested state before we even take a bite. To make things more difficult, often enzymes are not listed on food labels at all and instead fall under the category of "natural flavors." This is puzzling—after all, enzymes don't have flavors—but FDA regulations allow this. In this case, a protein powder that adds enzymes can disguise a process for creating free amino acids (including glutamate) by simply claiming it contains "natural flavors."

Manufacturers could easily report the level of free amino acids, short peptides, and intact protein in a protein powder, which would inform consumers of the amount of degraded protein in their products. But they don't.

Before I began my journey to understand the sources of free glutamate in the food supply, I didn't know how to interpret food ingredient labels—even with a PhD in biochemistry. But you don't have to be a biochemist to make healthy choices. As consumers, we can protect ourselves from ingesting excessive amounts of MSG. We do this through education and understanding the sources of MSG, the food manufacturing processes that generate it, and the many ways free glutamate can be labeled. Through our collective behaviors, we can make a difference in the food supply. We can communicate with our wallets that we only support products with transparent labels and ingredients that nourish, rather than make you sick.

Unblinding the Glutamate Obfuscation

Free glutamate goes by many names, and it is a component in at least 50 food additives, as shown in table 2.2. During my research, I was shocked to find out how long ago the many names for MSG were revealed and reported. As early as 1991, a *60 Minutes*[8] story exposed some of the alternative names for MSG, and so the practice of disguising MSG in food is certainly not breaking news. What is new is our knowledge of how excess glutamate in the food supply may be linked to America's current health crisis. Although the realities of obesity, addiction, diabetes, and myriad other health issues facing us today may seem insurmountable, one approach to these problems is plainly clear: eat more whole foods, and avoid overly processed foods. Keep reading!

To start, table 2.2 lists factory-processed food ingredients that can contain either hydrolyzed protein or free glutamate.

Table 2.2. Food Label Ingredients That Contain Glutamate

Accent®	Einkorn	Nori
Agar/Agar-Agar	Emmer	Nutrasweet®a
Ajinomoto	Enriched anything (e.g., vitamins, minerals, protein)	Nutritional yeast
Amino acid chelate (aspartatea, glutamate)	Enzyme modified/ containing enzymes	Oligodextrin
Annatto	Epicor®	Pea protein (isolates)
Artificial flavors	Extractsb (e.g., protein, mushroom, beet extracts)	Pectin
Aspartamea, aspartatea, aspartic acida	Farina	Potato flakes
Atta	Farro/faro	Protease (an enzyme that breaks protein bonds)
Autolyzed anythingb (e.g., autolyzed protein, yeast)	Fermented (e.g., grains, protein(s), soy)	Protein fortified
Barley (flakes, flour, malt, pearl)	Fertilizer	Protein powder
Bee pollen	Fish sauce	Protein solids
Beet (concentrate, juice, powder)	Flavor enhancer	Rice syrup
Bouillon	Flavors	Rye bread and flour
Breading (bread stuffing)	Fortifiedb (e.g., added vitamins, nutrients, protein, amino acids, minerals)	Seasoned salt
Brewers yeast	Fu (Japanese dried wheat gluten)	Seasoning(s)
Broth	Gelatin	Seaweed/seaweed extract
Brown rice syrup	Glutamate/Glutamic acid	Seitan

Table 2.2. Food Label Ingredients That Contain Glutamate (*continued*)

Bulgur	Gluten	Semolina
Calcium caseinate	Graham flour	Smoke flavoring(s)
Calcium glutamate	Gum (e.g., guar, xanthan)	Sodium caseinate (disodium caseinate)
Carrageenan	Hydrolyzed anything[b] (e.g., hydrolyzed oat flour, protein, vegetable protein)	Soup base
Casein/Caseinate	Isolates (protein isolates)	Soy (as in soy extract, protein, protein concentrate, isolate, sauce, and lecithin)
Cheese	Jerky	Spelt
Chicken/pork/beef "base" or "stock"	Kamut	Spice(s), Spice blends
Chicken/pork/beef "flavoring"	Kelp/kelp meal	Spirulina
Chlorella	Kombu/kombu extract	Splenda®
Chocolate liquor	Lipolyzed butter fat	Stock
Citrate/Citric acid	Low-/no fat	Sweet'N Low®
Coconut aminos (amino acids)	Magnesium glutamate	Tamari
Collagen (hydrolyzed collagen)	Malt (e.g., syrup, flavorings, flours)	Tangle extract
Corn (canned, starch, syrup, sugar, solids)	Maltodextrin	Textured protein
Cultures	Matzo, matzo meal	Tofu
Cured meat	Meat flavorings (chicken, beef etc.)	Tomato, processed (e.g., paste, powder, sundried)
Dehydrated egg	Milk byproducts (e.g., condensed, evaporated, whey)	Triticale

Table 2.2. Food Label Ingredients That Contain Glutamate (*continued*)

Dehydrated protein	Milk powder/reduced fat milk (lactose-free)	Ultra-pasteurized
Dextrose (using wheat, fermentation, or enzymes)	Miso	Umami
Disodium guanylate	Modified food starch	Vegetable gum
Disodium inosinate	Molasses	Vetsin
Dough conditioner(s)	Monoammonium glutamate	Vinegar (e.g., apple, balsamic, white, wine)
Dried peas	Monopotassium glutamate	Vital gluten
Dulse	Monosodium glutamate, MSG	Wheat (bran, flour, germ, starch)
Durum	Natrium glutamate	Whey (protein, concentrate, isolate)
Egg powder	Natural flavor(s)/ flavorings	Yeast[b] (e.g. extract, food, nutrient, paste)

[a] While not glutamate, these ingredients act like glutamate in the body.
[b] These ingredients are manufactured using a process that creates MSG.

As I compiled this list, what started as a hunch became a sobering reality: modern diets contain too much glutamate. In 1959, MSG received the GRAS (Generally Recognized As Safe) label from the FDA when, the statement goes, it is consumed at "customary levels." These customary levels have never been defined and, in the more than 60 years since this label was issued, the amount of free glutamate in our environment has increased over a thousandfold—at least. Not one MSG safety study examines chronic exposures to MSG at the level representative of today's diets. Yet an examination of the scientific literature leads one to the irrefutable conclusion that excess glutamate in the body is harmful.

Estimating just how much MSG the average person in industrialized nations consumes is challenging. For over 40 years, studies have attempted to estimate the amount of free glutamate in diets.[9] One of these studies was funded by a victim of Parkinson's disease, who likely had a personal reason for wanting more information regarding the levels of unlabeled MSG in foods. Researchers examining the effects of MSG often have to estimate the amounts in the diet to conduct meaningful studies. One 2010 study examining the effects of MSG on the vagus nerve (a critical branch of neural circuitry that basically connects our brain to our gut) estimated that the amount of MSG in the modern diet is 2 g/day.[10] Although this is nearly four times the amount of added MSG in food as estimated by the FDA, it is still much less than what consumers may actually be ingesting, as we shall see.

Further confusing consumers is inaccurate or, at the very least, misleading information by political interests and regulatory bodies. Here's a quote from the FDA website, which attempts to mitigate concerns about MSG levels in food: "a typical serving of a food with added MSG contains less than 1 gram of MSG."[11]

Another quote from the International Food Information Council (IFIC) touts why MSG isn't an issue and why there isn't much in the diet: "The average American consumes . . . less than 1 gram of glutamate per day from MSG."[12] Hard to believe, when there is enough pure MSG manufactured each year to feed every man, woman, and child on the planet 1.2 grams of MSG per day, and the number doesn't include the amount of MSG enriched in food as a result of commercial food processing.

Factory-Processed Foods: Do the Math

So how much MSG is the average person consuming every day if we add in the hidden sources? Is it enough to be significant? Using data that is freely available in the scientific literature, I have done the math. The amount of MSG an average person consumes, based on the published values for the known amount of processed food that is consumed per person, the average amount of protein in that food, and the extent to which that food is processed, is given in table 2.3. Spoiler alert: ultraprocessed food is the biggest source of MSG in modern diets.

Table 2.3. Estimated Daily Consumption of MSG in Modern Diets from Protein in Processed Food

Source of Glutamate	Amount Consumed (grams/day)
Group 1: Unprocessed or minimally processed foods (e.g., raw vegetables, nuts, meats, juices, flours, pasta, yogurt)	~0.5 g
Group 2: Processed culinary ingredients (e.g., oils, starches, syrups)	~0.1 g
Group 3: Processed foods (e.g., canned vegetables, bread, cured meats, cheese)	~1.5 g
Group 4: Ultraprocessed food products (e.g., canned pasta, snacks, frozen dinners, sweetened juices, breakfast cereals, infant formula, chicken nuggets, desserts)	~8.5 g

Note: NOVA classification of factory processed food was used to define food groups.
Source: Carlos Augusto Monteiro et al., "The UN Decade of Nutrition, the NOVA Food Classification and the Trouble with Ultra-Processing," *Public Health Nutrition* 21, no. 1 (March 21, 2017): 5–17, doi:10.1017/s1368980017000234.

The Takeaway

The numbers in table 2.3 are rounded for simplicity and their interpretation is straightforward. The largest amount of MSG in our diets—approximately 8.5 grams—comes from ultraprocessed food. This amount is simply created from the protein content of foods through the manufacturing *process*, not from MSG added as an ingredient by the manufacturer.

But MSG *is* being added, so the amounts of MSG in these food categories are certainly higher. From the list of ingredients that contain MSG presented in table 2.2, it is clear there are many other, hidden ways that MSG can be added to food that aren't indicated on the label. Remember, the amounts of MSG shown in table 2.3 doesn't include flavors, additives, enrichment with amino acids, or the many other common sources of MSG in our food.[13]

Also recall that more than 3.5 million metric tons of pure MSG is manufactured every year, and this ends up in the food supply. As described earlier in this chapter, this pure MSG is enough to feed each of the 8 billion people on Earth 1.2 grams of MSG per day. We know MSG is not being distributed equally to everyone; most of it is clearly finding its way into modern diets. For that reason, and for all the reasons given in the preceding paragraphs, I believe the numbers presented in table 2.3 are conservative and underestimate the amount of MSG consumed daily in modern diets. But even on face value, the average consumer in industrialized nations is easily consuming approximately 10 grams of free glutamate—daily! Some researchers have found that there can be close to 10 grams of MSG in a single dish, depending on the food culture. This observation was published over 30 years ago![14] The sobering fact is that the true amount of MSG ingested by modern consumers is undoubtedly higher than 10 grams per day.

Alarmingly, chronic long-term exposure to this amount of glutamate, ingested daily, has never been tested in animal safety studies. These data are nonexistent, but also alarming is the data we *do* have. There is abundant evidence from animal studies showing that acute (one-time) consumption or administration by injection of glutamate in the 0.5 g/kg range can cause severe neurological damage, particularly for young animals with developing brains.[15] That dose is equal to 1.5 g of glutamate for a 3 kg (6 lb, 10 oz) human infant, or 5 g of glutamate for a 10 kg (22 lb) toddler. Note that with older children—whose brains are still developing—5 to 10 grams of glutamate is an amount easily consumed from eating the foods kids find readily available. Suffice it to say, what we know—and what we don't know—about the effect of ingesting large quantities of MSG in humans is enough to suggest that today's modern diet, with its focus on processed and ultraprocessed foods, poses a fundamental health risk.

What's Next

To fully understand the issues and the evidence, in the following chapters I will explain how glutamate functions in the body, its role as a neurotransmitter, its role in disease, its relationship to inflammation, and how all of this is connected to the body's gut microbiome. Remember, the microorganisms that help us digest our food depend on the nutrients we serve them through our food choices. Our gut microbiome, in fact, is our partner in health. But we aren't eating for two—we're eating for trillions.

Taylor and I now eat a diet of fresh, organic, whole foods that I would not exchange for anything. I also recognize that a completely whole food diet still contains some free glutamate. That amount is not a problem for the vast majority of the population. There is an evolutionary purpose for the low levels of glutamate found in natural food. Glutamate in ripe fruits, nuts, and vegetables likely allowed our gatherer/wanderer ancestors to determine which foods were ripe enough to pick and eat. Glutamate also signals the presence of proteins, providing a good detection mechanism—and desire for—energy-rich foods necessary for survival.

As you will see in the rest of this book, glutamate in food performs essential physiological functions, such as telling the digestive tract how much protein to expect. It triggers digestive functions, such as activating taste receptors, motility in the intestine, and secretion of digestive enzymes.[16] This is how glutamate in food is supposed to work when the amount of glutamate you ingest is the amount found naturally in foods. Also in whole foods are the right proportions of proteins, fiber, fats, carbohydrates, vitamins, minerals, and many co-factors that aid in the metabolism of glutamate—a natural balance that is highly distorted in commercially processed foods.

The total free glutamate estimated in a whole food diet is between 0.5 gram and 1 gram per day, at least one order of magnitude less than the amounts found in the standard diets of our modernized civilization. That amount is enough to make food taste good. Homegrown tomatoes, famously yummy, contain glutamate. I find them to be delicious just the way nature made them.

So those are the numbers. In the next chapter I'll introduce you to the players, those powerful interests that are committed to keeping the amount of glutamate you are ingesting a secret.

3

Safety Concerns and Business Interests Collide

I WAS MAD. WHEN I STARTED MY DETECTIVE WORK TO LEARN WHAT exactly I was feeding my family, I kept asking myself, "How can the ingredients in the food we eat be such a mystery?" But when my sleuthing revealed what was actually in the jar or package on the grocery shelf, I became alarmed, and then angry. I had discovered that the food industry was feeding us vast amounts of MSG and doing their best to keep it a secret.

This revelation changed how I felt about the products I had previously believed in. The chain of trust, from manufacturer to grocer to consumer, relies on truth, but we have been deceived. There is no doubt that the young salesclerk at the natural foods store earnestly believes that the protein powder she is recommending will benefit your health. The health food store owner is confident he has done all his homework and may insist the umami flavoring he sells has little to do with MSG. Sadly, we have all been duped.

To see why so many people are blinded to the health risks posed by MSG and glutamate-enriched processed foods, we must go back in time. The debate regarding the safety of MSG began more than 65 years ago when, in 1957, a research team reported the toxic effect of MSG to the retina.[1] Many decades later, despite over 40,000 scientific publications authored by hundreds of researchers connecting retina damage (think macular degeneration) to glutamate toxicity, the association of this health ailment to MSG in food has never received the publicity it deserves. John Olney, medical doctor and professor of psychiatry, pathology, and immunology at Washington University School of Medicine, was an early pioneer demonstrating the toxic effects of MSG. He began publishing his findings in the late 1960s,[2] and continued publishing on the toxicity of glutamate for decades. He documented glutamate toxicity's associations with brain lesions, obesity, psychiatric disorders, and brain tumor growth.[3] He was the first to coin the term *excitotoxins*, and for over 30 years advocated for MSG's greater regulation in foods.

Nonetheless, in 1959—just two years after the first scientific studies began to raise safety concerns about MSG—the U.S. Food and Drug Administration classified MSG as GRAS (Generally Recognized As Safe).[4] This designation has never changed, despite all the research in the decades that followed that challenged this assumption, and the widely reported ill effects experienced by consumers. Much money has been spent to protect that safety classification. The factory-processed food industry is a trillion-dollar industry that has funded glutamate-related research and, today, through its various committees, populates World Health Organization (WHO) Codex Alimentarius Commission meetings, influencing food standards, codes of practice, and safety guidelines that specify all requirements related to foods around the world. Unfortunately, evidence suggests that food politics influence published nutritional information[5] and determine the standards for what defines nutrition.

The "Glutamate Is Safe" Debate Is Heavily Funded by the Food Industry

One of the biggest hurdles facing awareness of glutamate's effect on health is the unrelenting efforts of the glutamate industry to tout glutamate's safety and to discredit scientific research that suggests otherwise. Wait—a glutamate industry? You may be asking yourself, "why is there a glutamate industry, and what is it?" Here's the history.

In 1969, around the time there was increasing concern about MSG in food, the International Glutamate Technical Committee (IGTC) was formed to represent the interests of the glutamate industry. Food companies that have a vested interest in using the ingredient to enhance the flavors of their foods and make their foods addicting pay membership fees to IGTC. The IGTC then directly funds MSG research and the marketing of its safety. Among the committee's international members are many of the world's largest food companies. These companies are involved in such diverse areas as the manufacturing and marketing of food ingredients; spice and flavor blends; and canned, frozen, and other packaged processed foods.

In 1977, The Glutamate Association (TGA) was formed as a subsidiary of the IGTC to represent the U.S. food industry's interests in MSG. Both committees exist under the umbrella of the Robert H. Kellen Company. Who are they? The Kellen Company is also an umbrella for the International Food Additive Council (IFAC), which is governed by companies like Monsanto and Dupont. Through its lobbying efforts, the IFAC protects and advances the use of food additives.

The groups protecting the food supply status quo are many, and the glutamate industry's media and scientific publication systems are vast. When MSG is implicated in negative health effects, the glutamate industry is quick to respond. For example, the well-publicized Thai and Chinese population studies that linked MSG consumption to metabolic syndrome and obesity, respectively, and a German study that linked MSG consumption to obesity, excessive desire to eat, and short stature,[6] were quickly met with rebuttals published in non-peer-reviewed nutrition journals funded by the International Glutamate Technical Committee.[7]

Predictably, these rebuttals completely refuted the original studies' conclusions. A study funded by the glutamate industry also concluded that free glutamate in infant food was not deleterious to health,[8] allowing MSG to remain in infant foods, unlabeled. A glutamate industry–funded study concluded that, although the level of glutamate in the blood increased when subjects ingested glutamate in food, there was no ill effect.[9] IGTC, along with the National Institutes of Health (NIH), funded a study claiming that dietary glutamate does not activate the nervous system,[10] despite many studies showing otherwise. The upshot is the glutamate industry's response to scientific studies that they don't like is swift, and questions about glutamate's safety are overwhelmingly refuted by industry-sponsored studies that produce results favorable to the industry.

Have no doubt that Big Food is paying attention to what is being published. Take a quick glance at the masthead of nutrition journals such as the *American Society for Nutrition* and you'll see familiar names, including Abbott, Cargill, the Coca-Cola Company, the Dannon Company, DuPont, General Mills, Herbalife, Hillshire Brands Company, Kellogg, Kraft Foods, Mars Chocolate, McCormick, Monsanto, National Cattlemen's Beef Association, National Dairy Council, Nestle, PepsiCo, Pfizer, the Sugar Association, and Unilever. When Big Food is a proud sponsor of nutrition journals, the potential for the spread of misinformation is worrisome.

Case in point: Much of our knowledge with respect to the treatment and causes of obesity in humans stems from experiments with obese lab animals. For over 30 years, MSG has been used to create obese rats and mice in the lab to better understand how to treat obesity in humans. Despite over 30,000 scientific publications linking MSG to obesity, insulin and leptin resistance, and energy utilization disorders (more to come on this in chapter 7, "Glutamate and Disease"), these studies—because they use lab animals—are often discounted by the glutamate industry[11] as not representative of humans. Yet these same studies form the basis of preclinical trials for developing drugs to treat humans. They inform our understanding of obesity, diabetes, and other associated diseases that are part of the world's growing obesity health epidemic.[12] And we are asked to believe that the way scientists create obese rats—which is feeding them MSG-laden food—is unrelated to anything that could be causing the epidemic of obesity in modern civilizations. This, when we have witnessed a thousand-fold increase, at least, in the amount of MSG being added to the human food supply since the 1970s.

The food industry's attempts to obfuscate the connections between glutamate and obesity makes it difficult for researchers to use conventional thinking to explain why processed food (i.e., food enriched in glutamate) is fattening. Case in point is a 2019 study by researcher Kevin Hall at the National Institute of Diabetes and Digestive and

Kidney Diseases, an account of which appeared in the popular magazine *Scientific American*.[13] Hall led a study in which volunteers were kept in a hospital metabolic ward for four weeks. Participants were divided into two groups matched for age and gender and offered two different diets. The diets were matched for calories, fiber, carbohydrates, protein, fats, sugar, and sodium, but had this important difference: One group was given a diet of whole foods, with lots of vegetables, whole grains, and other unprocessed or minimally processed foods like roast beef, nuts, butter, and full-fat yogurt. The other group was offered ultraprocessed foods, which included processed cheese, hot dogs, canned ravioli, sugared cereals, margarine, and fruit-flavored drinks. All the meals contained twice as many calories as a person would need to maintain their body weight, and people were told to eat as much as or as little as they liked. They did this for two weeks and then the groups switched diets.

The results of the experiment were straightforward: in two weeks, individuals on the ultraprocessed food diet gained about two pounds, and those on the diet of whole foods lost about two pounds. Why? The explanation is that, even when the meals were matched for all the macronutrients, calories, and fiber, people eating the ultraprocessed food consumed an additional 500 calories a day, compared to their whole food–eating study mates. Simply put, people on the ultraprocessed food diet overate, every day. Clearly, the ingredients in ultraprocessed foods caused people to consume many more calories than they needed. (Lest you worry about folks getting fat as their reward for participating in this study, let me be quick to add that when the diets were switched, those who had gained the extra weight lost it, and those who lost weight gained it back, so at the end everyone came out about the same as when they started.)

Meanwhile, the MSG safety debate continues. But let's be clear: the glutamate industry has a loud voice, and it funds the effort to populate the scientific literature with studies touting glutamate's safety. There is far too much money circulating among food manufacturers, pharmaceutical companies, and medical industries for this to stop anytime soon. I thought about conducting a properly designed study myself to look at the effects of MSG in a chronically inflamed population, such as individuals with autism. What stopped me? Money. Studies cost money, and there is a great deal of bias involved in what research gets funded. Funding for such a study is still one goal for my nonprofit organization, Unblind My Mind.

That industry-funded research produces results favoring the funders is not new, and it is not limited to the glutamate industry. Unfortunately, the potential for research bias exists whenever a particular outcome is connected to a sponsor's profit (or a researcher's continuation of funding). Nowhere is this truer than in drug development. In pharmaceutical studies, positive results are four times more likely when the drug's manufacturer funds the study. With cancer drugs in particular, the likelihood of favorable results is eight times greater when companies producing the drug pay for studies, compared to when funding comes from an independent source.[14]

If you have any doubt about the ability and willingness of those with vested interests to pull out all the stops when it comes to obfuscation of scientific findings, read no further than *Merchants of Doubt: How a Handful of Scientists Obscured the Truth on Issues from Tobacco Smoke to Global Warming* by Naomi Oreskes and Erik M. Conway.[15] Think about it: if the tobacco industry with a toxic, deadly product can confuse the public with pseudo-science and sway public officials for decades, then we should be careful not to underestimate how food safety oversight is influenced by corporate interests.

Nonetheless, small studies examining the effects of MSG in specific ailments like fibromyalgia, headaches, liver inflammation, and dysplasia do exist.[16] It is not likely you have heard of them, as these never surface to mainstream news. Rather, they are lost in the sea of "science" publications funded by the IGTC and its many subsidiary committees. Trade advocacy groups can conduct larger and more costly studies, and industry-funded research can quickly refute, or even bury, the small science study that produces evidence that the food industry finds unfavorable.

I am not the only one who has noticed this. In my research, I have come across other individuals who have tried to raise public awareness of the health issues associated with MSG in the food supply. They have also written books and started organizations to raise awareness of the

MSG health issue.[17] There were even attempts for better ingredient labeling laws through citizen petitions to the FDA, which were denied.[18]

Once I was unblinded, I started to see all around me people whose health was seriously impacted by the foods they ate, and I struggled to find a way to share what I had learned. Then an opportunity presented itself, in the most unexpected way. It was July 4 and I was at the beach with Taylor. She struck up a friendship with a boy her age that was absolutely charming in its sweet innocence. As these five-year-olds held hands and climbed rocks together, the boy's father approached me and said, "Any child that can get my boy to climb rocks like that has a truly remarkable ability to connect." As we were chatting, I told him how Taylor, just a little over a year ago, would not socialize with any children. I told him of our journey, and he asked me if I had ever considered doing a Technology, Engineering, and Design (TED) talk. The truth is, I love speaking, and the thought that someday I might have the kind of public platform that TED provided was my dream. This man was a professional videographer, and in the end, he created a video of me walking through local grocery stores, translating ingredients on food labels for viewers. This kind person also helped me produce an audition video, which resulted in an invitation to give a TEDx talk. Such connections help shape my mission to build a community passionate about making a change to improve the health of a nation, one bite at a time.

Now let's get to the science and see what glutamate does in the body—and why too much glutamate in the diet is *excitatory*. Excited? Before you say yes, know that I don't mean that as a positive thing.

4

Overexcited

GLUTAMATE IN THE BODY

EVERY PARENT WANTS THEIR CHILD TO BE HAPPY. I CAN SAY ABSO-lutely, without equivocation, that when we changed our diet to REID, Taylor (and I) were happier—within days. Taylor had newfound delight in things that she had previously ignored or even despised. For the first time, she was open to interacting with us. I can only describe her as being *calmer in her body*. But there were bad days, too. When there was a significant food infraction, her reaction had all the earmarks of her suffering a "trauma" to the body. One event in particular stands out in my memory. Taylor was attending a company picnic with my husband (where monitoring of her food went by the wayside and she ate whatever she wanted). Once she came home, I observed she was trembling. Her lip was quivering and she was unable to calm herself. That night, her legs shook and she had night sweats. For the next three days, she cried over the smallest thing, a classic case of emotional dysregulation. I knew all those symptoms were brought on by exposure to excess glutamate. Neurologically, her cells were overexcited, her body and brain on fire.[1] She was traumatized.

Why do I refer to excess glutamate exposure as traumatizing? After all, in medical terms, trauma is usually associated with events such as not getting enough oxygen at birth, serious infections, and physical injury, like a blow to the head. But other, even more common things, like foods, can induce inflammation and trauma in the body. Such traumatic events are recorded in our neurological and immune memory and may manifest as prolonged fight/flight reactions (classic examples being anxiety, panic attacks, or generalized fear). Trauma can result in chronic immune activation (such as found in mast cell disorder,[2] autoimmune disease, and allergies). Excess glutamate inflicts trauma on the body in the form of protracted and unrelenting stress as the body tries to respond to excitatory stimuli. For some, like Taylor, it produces symptoms such as racing heart, sweating, and trembling.

We might think that a person could learn to avoid foods that caused such bad reactions, but it's not that easy. The excess glutamate in glutamate-fortified foods rewire taste preferences so that we literally become addicted to these products, even if their effects on how we feel later are highly unpleasant. With repeated exposure, these taste preferences become neurologically hardwired and hard to kick. Let me explain.

A Short Course in How Glutamate Functions in the Body

First and foremost, glutamate functions as a *neurotransmitter* in the body. You can liken a neurotransmitter to the messenger in a communication chain, where the messenger (glutamate) delivers a message to a cell by binding to the cell's glutamate receptors. This causes the cell to release some of its own stores of glutamate and—like a phone tree—those glutamate molecules bind to neighboring cells, relaying the message and causing those cells to release glutamate, and so on. The myriad signals that ensue between the cells in our bodies allow us to process and respond to information that we receive through our senses of touch, taste, sight, sound, and smell—what is collectively known as our sensory system. These signals orchestrate learning, memory, motor movement, and digestion. Glutamate signaling is so critical to all aspects of life that if I had to associate any single molecule with a so-called "spark of life," it would be glutamate.

And there's more. In addition to its role as a neurotransmitter, glutamate regulates many of the body's critical *metabolic* functions, such as those necessary for energy production. Glutamate's combined functions—neurotransmitter and metabolic regulator—puts this amino acid inside every cell in the body, in the blood, and in every fluid that bathes the brain, the gut, the skin, heart, muscles, and eyes.

So what happens when our cells are exposed to excess glutamate in the food we eat? Let's start with the fact that we don't need to get glutamate from food—our bodies produce all the glutamate we require. We synthesize the exact amounts of glutamate we need, where it is needed, when we need it. Because we don't require this amino acid from diet, glutamate is defined as a "nonessential amino acid," but there is nothing nonessential about the role of glutamate in the body. And for optimal health, our bodies require a well-regulated and balanced glutamate system, something our bodies have evolved to provide.

To understand how that system can get out of whack, we take a dive into the microscopic space between two nerve cells (figure 4.1). *Glutamate signaling* is the term used to describe how nerve cells (also called neurons) communicate with each other, and how the nervous system's electrical impulses propagate. In simple language, glutamate signaling works this way: something—a stimulus—triggers a nerve cell to release glutamate into the space between cells. This region of *extracellular space* (space outside the cell) is called the *synapse*. Glutamate travels from the nerve cell across the synapse to *glutamate receptors* on the surfaces of neighboring cells. This produces a change in those cells. In the case of a nerve cell, glutamate binding causes *ion channels*—tiny openings on the cell's surface—to open. Charged particles, such as Na^+ (sodium) and Ca^{+2} (calcium) ions, then flow into the cell. This is referred to as *excitatory signaling*, and results in an electrical wave propagating down the length of the nerve fiber. Put simply, glutamate activates the nerve cell. The cell that is activated then releases glutamate into the extracellular space near other cells, which then binds to glutamate receptors on the surfaces of those cells, and so on, in a cascade of events that we call nerve conduction. All this happens in nanoseconds. Literally, in the blink of an eye, millions of glutamate signaling events can transform the thought in your brain to the action of picking up a pencil on a table.

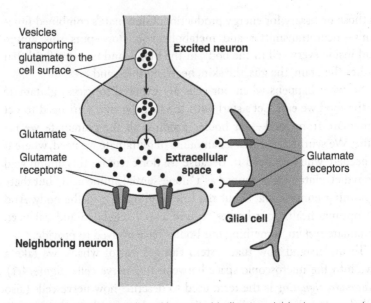

Figure 4.1 Glutamate signaling. Glutamate binding to neighboring neurons is the basis of nerve conduction. Note the presence of *glial cells*, which mop up excess glutamate if there is too much of it in the extracellular environment.

Glutamate isn't the only neurotransmitter in the body, but glutamate is unique in its sheer number of functions and versatility. Glutamate is the primary excitatory neurotransmitter in an estimated 40 percent of all neural signals conveyed by the body's nervous systems. It mediates 80–90 percent of the neural synapses in the brain's cerebral cortex, the largest part of the brain and the site of higher brain functions. But glutamate signaling in humans occurs throughout the entire body, wherever there are cells that contain glutamate receptors. In this way, glutamate's role is as diverse as the receptors it activates. In this receptor-activator role, glutamate acts like a single password that unlocks a wide array of cellular systems. Think of glutamate as a generalist, allowing the body to produce and regulate one chemical to carry out numerous and varied functions. This biological economy has a downside, however. The adverse effects of too much glutamate signaling—with diet being the root cause in many cases—impacts a huge number of systems, and that is why glutamate dysregulation has been linked to so many diseases. These diseases include Parkinson's disease, obesity, multiple sclerosis, Alzheimer's disease, and even addiction. Stay tuned; we will get to a discussion of these diseases in chapter 7, "Glutamate and Disease"— but first, let's get back to our primer on how glutamate functions in the body, and what happens when glutamate is not controlled.

Glutamate Excitotoxicity

One way to understand how too much glutamate in the body can be harmful is to remember that one of glutamate's functions is to excite the cell through electrochemical means. The body has protections to control the extent of glutamate signaling, but when these safeguards are rendered ineffective, too much glutamate can cause a cell to become *overexcited*. In other words, the cell keeps firing electrical charges. What happens when a neuron can't rest? Under a microscope, a neuron that has suffered the toxic effects of too much glutamate is easily recognized: it is swollen, and it is filled with an abnormal number of cellular structures akin to tiny, liquid-filled bubbles. These morphological changes are the visible evidence of *excitotoxicity*.[3] What is not visible through the microscope are the corresponding biochemical changes, which result in cell death. A cell can literally be excited to death by glutamate.

In a healthy person, glutamate performs its various functions, within nanoseconds if demanded, when its concentration inside and outside of cells is carefully controlled. The highest concentration of glutamate is inside brain cells, where it is an astonishing 5,000 to 20,000 times higher than it is outside the cell. If this amount of glutamate were to leak out of brain cells and into the extracellular fluid between neurons, the excitatory cascade that ensues could lead to a person's death. Brain cells manage such dangerously high concentrations of glutamate in two ways. First, brain cells store glutamate inside tiny cellular compartments called vesicles (see figure 4.1). This strategy keeps the cell's internal workings safe by locking away glutamate until it is needed. But that is not the only layer of protection brain cells have. The cell's thin membrane also acts as a barrier to keep glutamate inside the cell. You can think of the cell membrane as the "bag" that holds the cell's watery contents. In healthy brains, the cell membrane is sufficient to keep glutamate concentrations inside the cell extraordinarily high and keep the concentrations outside the cell exceptionally low.

Elsewhere in the body, glutamate concentrations fit the need. Blood, for example, can have glutamate concentrations a hundredfold higher than the brain's extracellular fluid. This could pose a danger if glutamate in blood leaked into the brain, but the brain has yet another barrier that protects it from excess glutamate. This is called the *blood-brain barrier*. The blood-brain barrier is a specialized array of cells and tissues that wrap the brain. In effect, the blood-brain barrier acts as a gatekeeper, allowing the blood to deliver necessary molecules like oxygen and glucose to the brain, while denying entry to other substances, such as bacteria or certain molecules, which might be harmful. Glutamate is one of the substances once believed to be stopped by the blood-brain barrier. However, there is evidence that this is not always the case. This is concerning. In order for our systems to work properly, the dramatic differences in glutamate concentrations found throughout the body must be maintained. Too much glutamate in the wrong place can be toxic, leading to overexcited cells, damaged neurons, and cell death.

Back in the 1960s, the very real specter of glutamate toxicity caused research scientist John Olney to coin the term *excitotoxin*. Olney observed that excess glutamate damaged the nervous systems of animals, particularly immature animals that were exposed to excess glutamate before the blood-brain barrier was fully developed. Olney applied the term excitotoxin to the amino acids glutamate, cysteine, and aspartate (used to make the artificial sweetener aspartame). By the 1980s, after years of study into the toxic effects of these amino acids, Olney's concern about the widespread use of glutamate and aspartate as food additives led him to issue the following warnings.

In 1984, Olney wrote:

> Evidence is reviewed supporting the view that excitotoxic food additives pose a significant hazard to the developing nervous system of young children. The following points are stressed:

1) although blood-brain barriers protect most central neurons from excitotoxins, certain brain regions lack such protection (a characteristic common to all vertebrate species);

2) regardless of species, it requires only a transient increase in blood excitotoxin levels for neurons in unprotected brain regions to be "silently" destroyed;

3) humans may be at particularly high risk for this kind of brain damage, since ingestion of a given amount of excitotoxin causes much higher blood excitotoxin levels in humans than in other species;

4) in addition to the heightened risk on a species basis, risk may be further increased for certain consumer sub-populations due to youth, disease or genetic factors;

5) despite these reasons for maintaining a wide margin of safety in the use of excitotoxins in foods, no safety margin is currently being observed, i.e., a comparative evaluation of animal (extensive) and human (limited) data supports the conclusion that excitotoxins, as used in foods today, may produce blood elevations high enough to cause damage to the nervous system of young children, damage which is not detectable at the time of occurrence but which may give rise to subtle disturbances in neuroendocrine function in adolescence and/or adulthood.[4]

These warnings did not result in any review of the safety of glutamate and aspartate by the FDA. Then, in 1988, John Olney wrote:

> Today we are witnessing an ironic situation; while knowledgeable neuroscientists are fervently attempting to develop methods for protecting CNS [Central Nervous System] neurons against the neurotoxic potential of endogenous Glu [glutamate] and Asp [aspartate], other elements of society are vigorously promoting unlimited use of exogenous Glu and Asp as food additives.[5]

Decades later, even more scientists are aware of the damaging effects of elevated glutamate, and Olney's "ironic situation" doesn't begin to describe the disconnect between current medical research and the glutamate industry's tactics in promoting glutamate in the food supply.

Now let's look at what happens on a molecular level when our bodies are exposed to high levels of glutamate and we experience an overexcited state.

The Advanced Course in Glutamate Excitotoxicity

While educating myself on the link between autism and diet, I found that one of the greatest sources for information and insight was the autism community itself. Parents in particular, motivated by the earnest desire to help the children they love, had educated themselves about autism, the central nervous system, glutamate signaling, and many of the topics I present in this book. When I spoke with parents about how some foods could be associated with autistic behaviors, I can only say that the level of understanding and scientific knowledge displayed by some of these parents was nothing short of remarkable. I am grateful for their input throughout this journey. This community's curiosity and persistent inquiries inspired my deep dive into the science. I cannot write this book without acknowledging this, and for that reason here is a more in-depth discussion about what I have learned, directed to those more knowledgeable readers, for whom the concept of glutamate signaling is old hat.

If you don't have the scientific background to understand what comes next, no worries. Just skip ahead to the next section. For those who *do* want to get into the nitty-gritty, well . . . hang on. Here we go!

Recall that glutamate signaling is triggered by an initial stimulus, which can be the taste of food, a painful injury, or the alarming sight of an advancing swarm of bees. The more "excitatory" the stimulus, the more glutamate signaling occurs, and the greater the number of neural pathways involved. It's as if one person shouts FIRE! in a crowded theater—others take up the call and shout FIRE! and in no time everyone is moving frantically for the exits. Glutamate signaling gets out the word that something is happening, and the body in return mounts a response proportional to the strength of the signal.

In truly dire situations, where survival requires that the body's neural response be prolonged and all-encompassing, a neuron would soon run out of available glutamate if the cell's metabolic machinery was not pressed into the service of making more. Glutamate synthesis is energetically costly to the cell, but when stressed it will make more glutamate, to the detriment of other cellular functions.

Take the brain, for example. The brain runs on glucose, a simple sugar. Brain cells convert glucose to energy in the form of ATP (adenosine triphosphate) using an efficient metabolic pathway called the citric acid cycle or Krebs cycle. When brain cells are overexcited and there is a great demand for glutamate, this pathway gets short-circuited. Need glutamate? No problem. The Krebs cycle in effect gets repurposed and glucose is shunted off to make more glutamate so that the brain can respond to the excitatory stimulus.

The important point is that glutamate signaling is energetically costly (calorie-wise) because using glucose to make glutamate competes directly with using glucose to make ATP (the energy molecule). In the case of the overexcited brain, the brain can become starved of energy needed for normal cellular functions. The shunting of the cell's resources away from energy production to glutamate production explains the sheer exhaustion a person experiences following an epileptic seizure. The abnormal firings of neurons and accompanying glutamate signaling simply drains the body of energy. Many of us have probably experienced fatigue due to prolonged periods of stress. I, too, would observe Taylor exhaust herself mentally and physically with her yes/no loops. For Taylor, there was no energy in her system for the normal development typical of a two- or three-year-old while these excitatory events were occurring. The glutamate signaling needed for neural development and learning was, in essence, being diverted to help the body survive the excitatory response being broadcast throughout her body.

The cell reacts in other ways to the rapid fire of excessive glutamate signaling. One of the consequences of excitotoxicity is *oxidative stress*. Oxidative stress results in an overproduction of extremely reactive molecules called free radicals, also called reactive oxygen species or ROS. ROS sport an unpaired electron and are very unstable, chemically speaking. They become stable by stealing an electron from another molecule, like DNA or an enzyme, which in turn can damage those molecules. ROS are a normal product of glutamate signaling and increase in concentration when cells are injured. If they get too plentiful, however, ROS can kill cells by damaging molecules that have important cellular functions. Fortunately, these potentially destructive free radicals are rendered harmless by micronutrients such as vitamins C and E, beta-carotene, and many other components of foods such as polyphenols and flavonoids—a topic I discuss in chapter 8. "Roadmap to Health: The REID Food Lifestyle." As you would expect, as the cell tries to protect itself from excitatory death, demand for these nutrients increases. If oxidative stress goes unchecked, however, cell damage, and cell death, follows.

The deleterious effects of excitotoxicity don't end with the death of the cell, which sounds bad enough. Upon death, the cell's contents—reactive metabolites, ROS, enzymes—spill into the extracellular fluid, where they can damage surrounding cells. What does the collateral damage look like? If a neighboring cell is only slightly damaged, its cell membrane may become less permeable and, in effect, close down. Nothing in or out. Further damage, and the cell membrane becomes ineffective as a barrier and the cell's contents leak out, creating more collateral damage.

Based on this mechanism of cell toxicity alone, it is no wonder that my daughter's exposure to the excitotoxic effects of excess glutamate in the food she ate made her agitated, afraid, and distraught. Physiologically, it amounted to trauma. Extrapolating from the cellular level, the case can be made that these excitotoxic effects spiral into what defines the majority of diseases plaguing modern societies, a case we will make in later chapters.

Wired: The Glutamate Receptor Map

What happens to cells that survive repeated excitotoxic assaults? Well, the body "learns" or trains from the experience. The number of glutamate receptors we possess on the surface of our cells is not static. Rather, it varies in a cell-specific manner as we age, and in response to our environment and experiences.[6] Not only do the number of glutamate receptor sites change, but also the receptor proteins themselves can be chemically altered as the result of events we experience.[7] All these changes form a meaningful record—you might say a memory, on a cellular level—of what a cell has experienced. There is a survival reason for keeping score. After all, glutamate signaling is used to regulate an amazing array of functions, including cognition, learning, behavior, movement, sensation, and all our recollections. Not surprisingly, the memory of trauma is recorded by our cells, as well.

Cells are not the whole story, though. When a person reacts to his or her environment, what's important is not individual cells but how those cells are "wired" together. If cells are bits of information, then neural networks are the delivery systems for sending that information to where it needs to go. Again, glutamate receptors account for 40 percent of all neural signals transmitted throughout our nervous system. In the brain it is much higher: more than 90 percent of synapses in the brain release glutamate. If you imagine the number and location of glutamate receptors in our bodies plotted on a map, such a map would be a fair proxy of the outlines of the body's nervous system. In effect, the glutamate receptor map traces the route traveled by a nerve impulse from the site of the original stimulus—a bee sting on a fingertip, say—to the brain, and then from the brain to the hand (which is quickly pulled back). As you might have predicted, experiences, as well as environment, can strengthen or weaken the connections in the glutamate receptor map.

In addition to the brain and nervous tissue, glutamate receptor maps have also been identified on organs and tissues such as the eyes, tongue, heart, pancreas, gastrointestinal tract, and skin where, in addition to their sensory and neural functions, they regulate cell metabolism. The upshot is that the body is constantly evaluating and responding to its environment, and that environment can be anything from blood sugar levels to the taste of a potato chip. All these reactions are mediated by glutamate, and if glutamate is out of whack, then these systems can be out of whack.

Wired for Glutamate? You Bet:
The Evolution of Taste Preferences

Evolutionarily, it makes sense that we would be wired for taste preferences. Nutrient- and energy-dense foods like ripe fruit and protein from any source are necessary for survival, and we should be driven to eat them. These healthy foods are also natural sources of glutamate, and so to further our species, humans have evolved an impressive set of taste receptors that light up when they detect glutamate in the food we eat. To start, each of us has a glutamate receptor map on our tongues, but it doesn't stop there.

Starting in 1990, researchers have been able to identify an entire array of glutamate-sensitive taste receptors extending from the mouth to the anus. It turns out that, hand in hand with the means to recognize nutritious food, Nature has wired us to seek it. If glutamate is detected along the digestive track, intestinal cells send a pleasure signal to the brain. This is not a trick to make us fat: given a choice, nature wants us to choose healthy, which means we have to *want* to eat healthy. Or better yet, *crave* nutrient-rich, energy-rich (i.e., glutamate-containing) foods. These cravings are not a problem when food is scarce, which has been the case throughout much of human history. When food is scarce, even if a person were drawn to the most tasty and ripest of what was available, there would be little chance of overeating.

We don't live in that world anymore.

In modern societies, the abundance of food is staggering. Because of supply chains that put fresh produce on grocery shelves in the dead of winter and Pacific salmon in shopping carts far from any ocean, the variety of food available to consumers is also unparalleled in history. So, what's for dinner? Food manufacturers want you to choose what *they* are selling, and unfortunately, they are adding excessive amounts of glutamate to foods that are not nutrient-dense or particularly good for us in order to hijack our palates. Such food is delicious and addicting.

I say addicting because the stimulation of glutamate receptors in the mouth trains the brain to seek those foods to repeat the pleasurable stimulation. Although this training served an evolutionary advantage in the past, today this reward system drives us to seek foods that have, as their primary attribute, the ability to stimulate our glutamate taste receptors. For the vast majority of people following the Standard American Diet (SAD), food preferences are determined by flavor preferences, rather than energy, nutrient, or caloric needs,[8] and with little consideration of health benefit. Our food choices are not a failure of character or education. Poor dietary choices are due, in large part, to a food industry that laces their products with glutamate to increase market share. The deck is stacked against us and we make food choices that are not in our best interests.

In addition to encouraging us to eat non-nutritious foods, another problem with fortifying foods with glutamate is that it sends false signals to the body, which reacts with inappropriate digestive responses. The taste receptors on your tongue have evolved to be sensitive to low levels of free glutamate, the amount found in natural, whole foods. When these taste receptors encounter the enriched concentrations of glutamate in processed foods, these receptors "misinterpret" the levels to mean that the food is protein- and energy-rich—and then signal the digestive tract and the brain to prepare the body for digestion of nutrients that may not be present. Over time, the disconnect between what the body expects and what it gets can lead to chronic diseases, such as diabetes. This is the topic of chapter 7.

When it comes to using this secret ingredient, manufacturers don't just enrich *food* with glutamate—they also put it in other products. Many oral care products such as toothpastes, mouthwashes, and dental floss, products used by dentists such as tooth polishes, and chewing gums contain glutamate in the form of flavorings. These oral products are not intended to be swallowed, and so target just the glutamate receptors on the tongue and soft palate of the mouth, with the goal of sending signals to the brain and forming positive associations with the products. Glutamate is also added to cosmetics, and body and skin care products, with the idea that absorption of even a small amount could stimulate glutamate receptors in the skin.

Creation of the Picky Eater

Food manufacturers understand clearly that glutamate is a potent tool for manipulating palatability in various foods. We can be trained to prefer glutamate as early as infancy by the addition of protein hydrolysates to infant formula. This training comes with significant implications for our metabolism, behaviors, and sensory signaling.[9] Once a preference for glutamate-fortified foods is established, unprocessed foods with natural (lower) levels of glutamate are rejected.

One common symptom of individuals with significant sensory dys-regulation is a narrow preference for foods. They are your classic "picky eater," with a list of food aversions that seems to include nearly all bitter, sour, and texture-rich natural whole foods. I work with many families in which the child has a self-limited diet heavily favoring non-nutrient foods (i.e., white, highly processed). In fact, we started our food journey with Taylor eating a very self-limited diet. I recall how just the sight of a green vegetable once caused such an uproar that one would think I had insulted her very being by suggesting such a food. Now I know there is a neurological and an evolutionary explanation to this behavior.

Failure to form positive associations to vegetables that are bitter, or nuts and seeds rich in texture, can create such powerful aversions to these foods that the body perceives them as toxic, especially if the taste receptors have been trained on factory-processed food.[10] In some families I have worked with, I've even encountered strong reflexes like gagging and vomiting when vegetables are initially introduced. While these unconscious reflexes are evolutionarily helpful and protect humans from ingesting toxic or spoiled food, it is challenging for a parent to convince a kid that dinnertime is not the time for that—no need to vomit, string beans are not poisonous!

Admittedly, once neurological preferences have been established for glutamate and sweets, the taste receptors need to be retrained before healthy eating is as rewarding as it should be. That is the fundamental concept behind the REID regimen—neurologically rewire the body, including the taste receptor map, from tongue to butt. While the success of taste receptor retraining may seem self-evident to anyone who has tried to eat more healthily, it is also supported by scientific data from animal feeding behavior studies.[11] Better food choices come naturally after taste retraining. Only by repeat exposures to nutrient-rich foods, while eliminating the processed foods that satiate the palate with flavor enhancers, will habits and preferences change. Rewiring the taste receptor map is the first step to recovering health.

5

The Microbiome

MEET THE REST OF YOUR BODY

AN EARLIER TITLE OF THIS BOOK WAS *A GUT FEELING*. WHEN I started writing it, the gut feeling I was referring to was the series of hunches that led me to discover that my daughter's autistic symptoms were managed with a REID food lifestyle. As I continued my research, "gut feeling" took on a whole new meaning. How we feel, and our health overall, is strongly influenced by the communities of micro-organisms that colonize our guts. How does this relate to our story about glutamate? The microbes in our intestines manufacture gluta-mate and other neurotransmitters as a way of communicating with us, their human host. Although they reside in our gastrointestinal tract, the communication networks of gut microbes extend to our brain, im-mune system, and beyond, and a diet of processed food affects them, too. Like humans, these microbes prefer certain foods. They are also capable of signaling to our brains that we should eat foods that benefit them, which is not necessarily food that benefits us.

When we eat, we feed the inhabitants of our gastrointestinal tract. *What* we eat determines which communities of microbes thrive or die, who gains influence, and who are resigned to be bit players in our gut's ecosystem. As in all life-or-death choices, we need to feed our gut eco-system wisely. We and our teaming trillions of tiny companions are partners for life, in sickness and in health.

The idea that our gut microbiota constitutes a complex ecosystem that can be damaged by our food choices is a relatively new concept in medical science. Scientists refer to these communities of microorganisms as the *microbiome*, and entire books have been written on the subject.[1] In this chapter, I'll introduce you to your microbiome, describe its role in health and disease, and discuss how different foods drive the microbiome to produce chemicals—including glutamate—that impact our health. First, let's start with some basics.

Human Microbiome

The human body is a big house hosting an estimated 100 trillion microorganisms. These single-celled organisms are collectively referred to as our microbiome, or sometimes our *microflora* or *microbiota*, and they are just as much a part of our human ecosystem as are the skin cells on our fingertips (which are themselves hosts to microbes). Like ecosystems everywhere, microbial communities in the gut form complex food webs and establish *trophic levels*, in which the waste products of one group of microorganisms provide food for others, which in turn break down the food further to provide food for the next level of microbes, and so on.

Human cells have a place in these trophic levels, too. In addition to their familiar job of absorbing the nutrients in food, human cells lining the intestine also absorb chemicals produced by microbial metabolism—microbial byproducts—which are called *metabolites*. One important metabolite produced by microbial action in the gut is vitamin B12, which is critical for human health. As we will see, however, our microbiome contains not just good residents. There are also the so-so, bad, and really *nasty* residents, too.

In addition to forming trophic levels, the microbiome behaves like an ecosystem in other respects. In the same way organisms everywhere vie for resources and seek competitive advantages, microbes in the gut compete for space and nutrients, sometimes producing toxins that kill off their competitors. There's also strength in numbers. These single-celled organisms can communicate with other similar gut microbes, and together act like a complex, large multicellular organism in our digestive tract. And like all living communities, microbial and human populations evolve together over time. Think about that—if we change, they change, and vice versa.

Earth ecosystems are classified according to location (i.e., wetland, tundra, deep sea), and our bodies' communities of microflora are no different. Our skin microbiome differs from our genital microbiome, which is different from our oral and gut microbiomes. Remarkably, the human gut microbiota is the densest ecosystem in the world and is estimated to consist of 10^{14} bacteria, viruses, fungi, and archaea (ancient single-celled microorganisms). At the time of this writing, researchers have identified approximately 1,100 species of gut bacteria organisms in human populations, with approximately 160 or so species living in the gut of any individual.

Let's take a tour of our intestinal tract (figure 5.1) and meet some of the residents.

Human Gastrointestinal Tract

Mouth

Approximately one-quarter of the total microbial population associated with the human body is found in the mouth. The microbes found in the biofilm coating your teeth (your dentist calls this plaque) are different from the microbes populating your gums, or those found in your saliva, cheek mucosa, or growing on your throat and tonsils.[2] Diet strongly influences the microbial composition of the mouth. In comparing the diet of a hunter-gatherer to modern industrial diets, pathogenic (disease-causing) bacteria are associated with the latter. While an increase in refined sugars in the industrial diet is part of the story connecting diet with disease (tooth decay comes to mind), glutamate-linked changes in the mouth microbiome also play a role in our health.

As described in the previous chapter, you might recall that in the 1990s researchers discovered the existence of a vast network of glutamate receptors, referred to as a *glutamatergic network*, in our digestive tract, stretching from our mouth to our anus. The food and oral

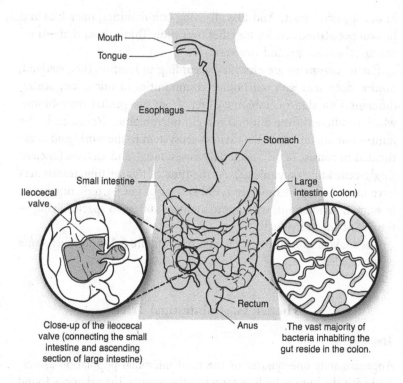

Figure 5.1 The human gastrointestinal tract. Glutamate taste receptors line the entire GI tract.

product industries took advantage of this discovery and today fortify products with glutamate to manipulate consumer preferences. The rationale is simple: the grocery aisle is crowded, and if adding glutamate to a product will boost sales, manufacturers see no reason not to do it. There is no regulation stopping them. But what we don't know *can* hurt us. The addition of glutamate drives our preferences to foods and oral products that satisfy flavor preferences, rather than satisfying our basic needs for energy and nutrients, or the imperative to avoid toxins.[3] These preferences translate into human behaviors that impact the makeup of our mouth microbiota.

To gain insight into the effects of glutamate on mouth microbes, I cite a study that measured the pathogenicity of a bacterium associated with periodontal disease, *Porphyromonas gingivalis* (formerly *Bacteroides gingivalis*). This bacterium becomes more virulent in the presence of protein hydrolysates (short peptides) that contain glutamate and aspartate.[4] These protein hydrolysates are abundant in processed foods, and so it is not a stretch to conclude that processed foods increase pathogenicity of this oral microbe. This promotes periodontal disease, which is characterized by gum inflammation and abscesses.

In another study with rats, the effect of a two-month exposure to MSG (1 percent and 2 percent solutions) on the oral mucosa was examined.[5] Compared to the control group with no MSG, both groups receiving doses of MSG displayed evidence of damage to cellular DNA and other tissue abnormalities. These changes were consistent with changes seen in precancerous lesions affecting various organs, including those associated with cancer of the mouth.

Based on studies like these, you might ask yourself why the food industry asserts there is no harm in fortifying products with a "natural" substance like glutamate. Evidence suggests otherwise.

Stomach

Long believed to be sterile, the stomach harbors a unique microbial environment which is distinct from other sections of the gastrointestinal (GI) tract because of its acidity (note that the acidity of gastric acid approaches that of battery acid). This keeps microbial populations low. When microbial metabolites created in the mouth (for example, nitrite from *Lactobacillus*) enter the low pH conditions of the stomach, they form new chemicals with antimicrobial properties, which also keeps microbes in check. Both conditions effectively discourage mouth microbes that are swallowed from colonizing the stomach and traveling into the intestine. Due to the challenges of studying microbial ecosystems within the stomach, though, not much is known about stomach microbes, with the exception of pathogenic bacteria like the ulcer-causing *Helicobacter pylori*.

Small Intestine

The same thing that makes the small intestine ideally suited for absorption of nutrients makes it ideal territory for microbial living: it has a lot of surface area, and it is sculpted with folds and finger-like protrusions that permit close physical contact between microbes and human cells. Stretched out and flattened, the inner lining of the small intestine, called the *mucosa*, has the surface area of a tennis court.

The small intestine is where human cells absorb most of the products of digestion. The microbiota, living on the surface of the intestinal wall and attached to food particles, helps this process by chomping down on otherwise indigestible foodstuffs and releasing more palatable molecules that its human host can absorb. The generalized term for this microbial metabolism, which occurs in the absence of oxygen, is *fermentation*. The microbes must work quickly, though. Half the contents of the small intestine will transit the entire small intestine in just two and a half to three hours.

Large Intestine

Next stop is the large intestine, which is mostly made up of the colon. Before we can move into the large intestine, though, we are stopped by the ileocecal valve, a circular sphincter muscle that squeezes tight to keep the contents of the upper large intestine from backflowing into the small intestine. Like any physical land barrier separating two communities (think of a mountain), the strategically placed ileocecal valve separates the microbial populations inhabiting the small and large intestines. And the two communities are quite different, both in terms of species makeup and numbers. Whereas the small intestine hosts up to 1000 bacteria per milliliter of volume (1 ml is equal to about 20 drops of liquid), the vast majority of the gut microflora—an astonishing 100 *billion* per milliliter of volume—reside in the colon. Here we find the bacterial workhorses of digestion, tasked with extracting nutrients from the leftover remnants from the upper GI that enter the lower GI. The bulk of this material is fiber—or I should say, the bulk of the material *should* be fiber. I'm not talking about fiber that is in a capsule or a powder in a container, but fiber that is contained in unprocessed whole food, particularly fiber from vegetables.

All this food transit stuff takes time. Although the large intestine is only one-quarter the length of the small intestine, transit through the colon is slow, typically requiring 30 to 40 hours.

The microbiota of the large intestine are essential for human life, and that is no hyperbole. We need them, and they like us, too. Every square inch of the colon intestinal wall teems with a diverse collection of necessary microbes: cellular energy producers, vitamin and co-factor synthesizers, neurotransmitter makers, and much more. These gut microorganisms not only produce substances essential to human cells, they also provide a line of defense against outside pathogenic invaders that would otherwise take over. Bacteria that have colonized our insides don't give up their seat at the table easily. They out-compete and out-eat (i.e., out-ferment) their rivals, sometimes even producing chemicals that function as antibiotics, targeting bacteria that are competitors or don't belong, or at least, are not welcomed as neighbors.

Although the small and large intestines support different microbial ecosystems, these ecosystems by necessity interact with each other. That is because when one microbial community eats, it releases nutrients that nourish the next, thus enabling a flow of nutrients from one set of microbes to the next. And along the way, our microflora feed *us* by releasing essential metabolites that human cells lining our intestine wall eagerly metabolize for energy. This completes the final loop in the greater human–microbiome ecosystem: humans provide the real estate and food, and the gut microbiome provides digestive functions, essential vitamins, critical neurotransmitters, hormones, and chemical regulators for human metabolism. In a balanced ecosystem, bacterial populations stay in check, inhabitants do their job, and both the gut microbiome and its human host prosper. I say bacterial because that taxonomic kingdom has been studied most. Viral, fungal, and archaea are part of the microbiome, too, and we are still gaining an understanding of their role in health and disease. What is clear, though, is that the human–gut microbiome connection is so close and necessary that some scientists refer to us and our microbial pals as a human *supraorganism*.[6]

Okay, that's the happily-ever-after version. Balance and harmony in the gut is definitely not what we are seeing today in the majority of the population, and evidence suggests that the modern diet and the preponderance of processed food is to blame.

Too Much of a Good Thing

Think of today's highly processed, manufactured food as being predigested. Processed and ultraprocessed foods are typically low in fiber, and enriched in fragmented proteins (short peptides), amino acids (glutamate in particular), sugars (the breakdown product of complex carbohydrates), and short-chain fatty acids (the breakdown product of fat). When these processed foods exit the stomach and hit the small intestine, microbes on the receiving end become lazy eaters, shutting off genes and unused metabolic pathways. And why not? Nutrients are plentiful and packaged into ready-to-consume pieces. Add a multivitamin to your routine and these microbes are living on easy street, thriving in the small intestine and increasing their colony size. Human cells easily absorb what they need, and our bacterial pals feast on quick meals without the energetically costly work of breaking down complex molecules such as flavonoids and polyphenols. The *cooperative* strategy of one group of microbes "cross-feeding" another group with the products of its digestion falls apart. Now key to surviving are *competitive* strategies, as everybody scrambles for the same ready-to-eat meals.

So, if food is about energy, why isn't pumping the body with amino acids, fatty acids, and sugar healthy for the human–microbiome ecosystem? This is more than just about calories. An analogy would be a pond ecosystem spiked with excess nitrogen and phosphorous from fertilizer runoff. With warm weather and lots of sun, algae in the pond have the opportunity for explosive growth, which in turn depletes the pond of vital substances like dissolved oxygen. The algal bloom also produces an excess of metabolites that are toxic to other inhabitants, like fish and frogs. Plenty of energy is provided to the ecosystem, but the readily available supply of nutrients provides an advantage to only a few species, and results in the death of others. Left unchecked, algae will become the dominant species and eventually suffocate and poison the pond, killing the ecosystem. A similar phenomenon commonly happens in the human gut ecosystem.

Community Diversity and Gut Health

One of the characteristics of a robust and resilient ecosystem is population diversity. Many of the same rules that govern the health of a pond apply to our gut. Diversity in the gut microbiome keeps microbial communities balanced. The reason processed and ultraprocessed foods deprive the human GI tract of microbial abundance and diversity is because they don't contain the complex molecules found in natural whole foods. Processed foods bypass the ordered trophic levels by which large molecules are broken down into smaller molecules, and the result can be an overgrowth of some microbes at the expense of others.[7]

The result of microbial imbalance is not just a toxic environment for our gut microbiome. Human health suffers as well.

To understand how human health depends on gut microbiome health, consider how your *intestinal mucosa* (the thin sheath of human cells lining the intestinal wall) is both a barrier and a port of entry. The mucosa layer is a port of entry because the human cells in the mucosa absorb nutrients from the intestinal contents, and these nutrients ultimately feed all the cells in the body. But the intestinal mucosa is also a barrier, keeping bad things out—things like pathogenic bacteria, toxins, viruses, and other infectious agents that would invade our bodies and do harm. A healthy microbiome helps maintain the integrity of this barrier by making metabolites needed by human mucosal cells. In addition, microbes in a healthy microbiome consume what we'll simply call "bad" metabolites, chemicals that are toxic to cells. When this doesn't happen, toxins can build up. Human cells become stressed because they aren't receiving the necessary nutrients and are expending energy dealing with toxins. The cells of the intestinal mucosa can lose function, and the result is erosion of the intestinal wall and its protections.

What does this look like? With erosion of the intestinal wall, the once-protective barrier becomes permeable and can no longer keep microbial and food waste products from entering the blood. Disorders like inflammatory bowel disease and irritable bowel syndrome (commonly referred to together as IBD and IBS, respectively), Crohn's disease, and diverticulitis are more common during this state. Autoimmune diseases, chronic immune activation, and energy utilization disorders like diabetes, obesity, and so many more are also believed to arise in this manner. This barrier permeability is what people mean by a "leaky" gut. In the worst cases, the gates open to an army of microbes looking to take advantage, allowing them to enter the bloodstream and cause infections elsewhere in the body. Infections of this type can lead to deadly sepsis, which occurs when the body's massive inflammatory response results in tissue damage and organ failure.

The connection between disease and an imbalance in the gut microbiome has been established in countless studies. For example, the hallmark of a multitude of nonspecific gastrointestinal symptoms such as chronic abdominal pain and bloating, diarrhea, and constipation is greatly reduced diversity in the gut microbiome. One consequence of reduced diversity is bacterial overgrowth, particularly in the small intestine. This may seem counterintuitive, but when the ecosystem is missing key players to keep the checks and balances, a few species will rule the region. This bacterial overgrowth is associated with so many illnesses that it has its own acronym: SIBO, for small intestine bacterial overgrowth. SIBO is diagnosed when your population of bacterial guests approaches millions instead of the tamer gathering of thousands.[8] Essentially, there's a party going on in the small intestine, creating so much metabolic waste and gas that the human host often experiences bloating, constipation and, in some cases, diarrhea. SIBO's one defining characteristic is that in a majority of cases, there is little diversity of species. The take-home message is that microbial diversity is associated with health, and lack of diversity is associated with sickness.

So what microbial species and communities *should* you have for an optimal microbiome? One thing that has made the human-microbiome wellness puzzle hard to put together is the fact that two perfectly healthy people can have very different microbiomes. Why is that? We are familiar with the idea that the particular species that make up healthy ecosystems can differ, and the human microbiome is no exception. Every human ecosystem is unique, defined by an individual's experience, which we call life. Encounters and competition throughout life determine which microbes stay or go. For that reason, the particular microbial species that join us at the table and dine on our daily meals can vary from person to person. This is the ecological reason why, of the approximately 1,100 species of gut bacteria found in human populations, only 160 or so such species live in the gut of any individual. As I'll describe in the final chapter of this book, by eating the right foods, you can make your unique 160 species work for you, not make you sick.

Birth of the Microbiome

We receive our first set of microflora from our mothers at birth, and likely before birth through the placenta.[9] Initially, an infant's microbiome is sparsely populated, reflecting what the newborn received from its mother and the immediate environment. However, this changes quickly, and what babies are fed makes a difference. By three to six weeks of age, analyses of fecal samples already show differences between breast-fed versus formula-fed infants. The breast-fed infants' microbiomes have a preponderance of bacteria that sets up the developing intestinal tract for carbohydrate metabolism, whereas the formula-fed babies' microbiome is geared toward fat and protein metabolism.

When children start to eat the same foods as adults by the end of their first year, their microbiome shifts to more resemble the adult microbiome. Adult microbiomes vary within populations and become more stable as we age, but across geographic regions, the makeup of the microbiome is highly influenced by diet. For example, a study showed that African children consuming a predominantly vegetarian diet rich in starch, fiber, and plant polysaccharides and low in fat and animal protein had significantly different microbial species in their microbiome than European children who had a diet high in animal protein, fat, sugar, and starch, but low in fiber.[10] Pathogenic bacteria were also found to be far less abundant in African study participants than in Western study participants. Here I am making the point that diet highly influences the microbiome—a theme I return to throughout this book.

Perhaps one of the most amazing things about the gut microbiota in newborns is that the first species of bacteria arriving on the scene "teach" the baby's immature immune system to accept their presence. This immune training is important because later on, as the immune system matures, it will learn to attack infectious bacteria, viruses, and other pathogenic agents without harming human cells. Our immune system does this using an elaborate chemical identification protocol that tags anything not derived from its own tissues as "foreign" and therefore potentially dangerous. To protect themselves from attack, early microbial colonizers immediately instruct the baby's developing immune system to accept their foreign microbial cells as human. That means that, while later the immune system may wage war against other bacterial invaders, "friendly" gut bacteria can peacefully coexist with the human cells in the intestinal mucosa. The body treats them as "self," the same as human cells, as these friendly bacteria aid digestion, churn out vitamins and metabolites, and generally make themselves useful. Human supraorganism, indeed!

The Human Microbiome Project

Much of what we know about the human microbiome began with the launch of the Human Microbiome Project in 2007. At that time, researchers were already reaping the benefits of the project's predecessor, the Human Genome Project, which envisioned mapping all of our human genes and their functions to discover the genetic links to health and disease. However, one of the outcomes of the Human Genome Project was surprising. A piece seemed to be missing—the human genome had far fewer genes than expected, given the complexity of humans.

To more fully understand the genetics of human health, researchers realized they needed to expand their view to include what they called the "microbial components of the human genetic and metabolic landscape."[11] In other words, human health was inexorably linked not just to human genes, but to the genes contained in the trillions of cells that made up the human microbiome. To give some perspective as to how much these microbial inhabitants contribute to our genetic composition, there are about 30,000 genes in the human genome and about 3 *million* in the microbiome. That's 99 percent of our combined genetic makeup! The Human Microbiome Project clearly established that the human body hosts a varied and vast microbial ecosystem, and that the proper metabolic functioning of these microbes was inextricably connected to human health.

Genetic sequencing of the human microbiome has also allowed scientists to examine differences in the bacteria microbiome correlated with sex, age, longevity, and types of chronic illnesses. The results are intriguing. For example, a whopping 400 genes (give or take a few) involving bacterial cell metabolism are altered in the gut microbiome of obese individuals, as compared to those of their more lean study partners.[12] Note that it is *bacterial* genes that make the difference in obese individuals—not human genes.

Although intuitively we understand that healthy microbiomes and healthy humans go hand in hand, the focus of current research is to define what constitutes healthy and unhealthy human–microbiome ecosystems. The data are coming quickly, and the rest of this chapter describes some of what we know so far and the glutamate–microbial connection to diet.

Processed Food: Microbial Metabolism and Glutamate Load

Evolutionary biologists have long postulated that, a million years or so ago, the control of fire and the advent of cooking our food led to profound changes in both the physical anatomy of our digestive tract and the composition of our gut microbiome. The modern diet, with its dependence on ever more processed food, has also changed the human gut microbiome composition in measurable ways. This genetic shift in the microbiome is associated with the current health crisis, which is characterized by the explosion of chronic diseases such as obesity, diabetes, IBS, generalized inflammation, and even chronic pain, as well as disorders impacting the brain such as dementia, depression, anxiety, addiction, autism, and other childhood developmental disorders.

Let's connect the dots between diet, our microbiome, and health, starting with what we know. The microbiome and its proper function are dependent on the host diet.[13] This is undisputed. As compared to healthy individuals, a recurring theme in many cases of individuals suffering from chronic illnesses is a shift in microbial species inhabiting the gut and a corresponding shift in the metabolites these species produce. This observation has been thoroughly documented with regard to many chronic illnesses, including those that impact the brain and cause negative behaviors and emotions.[14]

We also know that, with such a milieu of chemicals produced by the trillions of organisms inhabiting our gut, chemical imbalances can ensue when things go awry. At this point in my career, I have reviewed thousands of metabolic and microbiome panels, and I can see how human metabolic test results can be influenced by microbial metabolism in the gut. Imbalances in the gut can be toxic to the host—and remember, the host is us.[15] On the cellular level, toxicity is defined as the point at which the human cell is no longer functioning optimally because the concentration of the microbe metabolite exceeds what the cell can utilize, eliminate, or neutralize. At toxic levels, the metabolite taxes the energy and function of the cell. Sure, we all have detoxification pathways to eliminate the toxins we are exposed to, but each of us has an individual threshold above which our health becomes impacted. This point can't be overemphasized: the threshold at which *chemical imbalance* becomes *chemical toxicity* is most certainly different for different individuals, depending on a person's genetic susceptibility, history of other toxic exposures, and overall health. Toxicity? Everyone takes this personally.

The third piece of evidence connecting diet with an unhealthy microbiome gets back to glutamate. Glutamate, our trustworthy chemical messenger, is tasked with sensing and reporting on the state of the environment, whatever that may be. Of course, in the intestine, the contents of the gut *is* the environment, and one of the most interesting things cells in your gut tell your body is what you ate today. Information about a food's nutritional and caloric composition allows the body to adjust appetite hormone levels, among other things, and tells you that you have had enough to eat . . . or urges you to eat more. Glutamate signaling also informs the body if the gut contents are toxic. In this case, you may get the message, "eject contents!" triggering the vomit reflex, or alternatively, diarrhea.

The relationship between consumption of excess glutamate, a disrupted microbiome, and disease can be inferred from numerous human and animal studies. The take-home is that different species of gut microbes become more abundant when humans or animals are fed glutamate-enriched diets.[16] The abundance of these microbes is correlated with higher concentrations of glutamate in the blood.[17] In fact, elevated concentrations of glutamate in the blood is the single most strongly correlated metabolite found in one group of patients in particular. What disease do these patients have? The study I am citing looked at obesity,[18] which is affecting more and more individuals who consume modern diets.

Up to this point, we have been describing our gut microbiota as necessary and fundamentally *friendly* members of our human microbiome ecosystem. Although it's a pleasant exercise to imagine these microorganisms as stalwart partners in human health, the truth is, the microbes we host are devoid of loyalties beyond ensuring their own survival. With short reproductive cycles—around 20 minutes long—they can quickly evolve and adapt to changes in the environment, and that they do, adjusting gene expression, metabolism, and species abundance to fit the nutrients supplied. For example, if there is a lot of glutamate in the food being delivered to our gut microbes, these microorganisms adjust their metabolism to utilize glutamate, and in the process create an ecosystem thriving on glutamate metabolism.[19] I'll talk more about this later in the chapter, but the point is that a gut microbiome fed excess glutamate looks very different from a "normal" gut ecosystem, with statistically significant increases in the abundance of some microbes over others.

The thing to remember is that, as in any ecosystem, when our gut microbiome is disturbed by disease or a significant change in the nutrient supply, stability gives way to disruption. This in turn gives rise to new microbial winners and losers. Researchers have documented that, given the opportunity, bacteria will overgrow and create imbalances,[20] a condition called "dysbiosis." Pathogenic bacteria, or even just ordinary bacteria, fight to gain a foothold in the disrupted landscape by competing for resources in ways we are just beginning to understand.

Gut Feeling: Modern Diets and the Microbiome

Have you ever consumed a meal that you later associated with feeling depressed, anxious, or irritable? These symptoms may very well have been the excitotoxic effects of the food on your cells.

Before I began our dietary journey, Taylor would eat only about five foods, all moderately to highly processed. What she ate—bagels and cream cheese, pizza, macaroni and cheese, pasta with butter or marinara sauce—was typical of the Standard American Diet (SAD). The connection between gut and brain became very clear to me as I observed Taylor's behavior drastically change after I removed processed foods from the menu. Not only was her emotional state better, it was as if her microbiome had undergone a "turnover" event and there was an entirely new bacterial crew at work, filling metabolic roles that had been abandoned by their predecessors. No longer did she experience bloating, constipation, and strong cravings for sugar. I also experienced firsthand how getting rid of processed foods positively impacted my own mood, energy, GI function, and so much more. After the whole family started eating better, I even could tell when my husband Mitch "cheated," as the irritability and depression was visible on his face after what we call a food infraction, which could have been as seemingly innocent as ordering a big burrito for lunch or having restaurant salad dressing on his salad.

I understand now that the behavioral and emotional improvements I observed were a function of improved metabolic balance, which was happening inside all our cells, the human ones and the trillions of microorganism cells making and consuming metabolites in our gut.

Unfortunately, simply labeling glutamate in food is not going to solve our food-related health problems. We know that the food industry cannot be trusted to provide foods that are truly healthy, as often advertised, and hidden glutamate in the food supply is hardly the only villain. To avoid a stress response from glutamate we need to consider the entire gut microbiome: what these microbes need to thrive, how and where they interact with human cells, and how this contributes to our overall glutamate load.

In this context, we see that the modern diet and the preponderance of processed foods are the real villains robbing us of our health because of the harm they do to our microbiome. Most of the foods on grocery shelves today do not deliver nourishment to the colon, where the vast majority of gut microbes live and work. Unfortunately, the consequences of starving this vital ecosystem are evident in the (literally) thousands of microbiome studies published yearly.

Let's take a specific example and drill down to see what is going on in light of what we've learned about the human microbiome ecosystem.

About 75 percent of the food in the modern diet is of limited or no benefit to the microbiota in the large intestine, and that is no exaggeration. The commercial processing of foods breaks down nutrients even before digestion begins, and these refined macronutrients—sugars, amino acids, fatty acids, and nucleotides—are almost entirely absorbed in the small intestine. What eventually reaches the large intestine is of limited value, as it contains only small amounts of the minerals, vitamins, and other nutrients necessary for maintaining this niche of the microbiota ecosystem. Fiber, the preferred food of the colon microbiota, is in woefully short supply in modern diets. On the other hand, protein, usually animal protein, is abundant.

What happens if you don't eat many fiber- and nutrient-rich foods? In this case, protein will be in excess relative to fiber in the large intestine, meaning this environment will favor protein fermentation. The adage "you are what you eat" is never truer than when considering the multitudes of microbial cells that form our microbiome. One class of bacteria that thrives on protein metabolism is *Clostridia*. This order of bacteria has many notorious members that are responsible for life-threatening illnesses, such as *C. tetani* (tetanus), *C. botulinum* (botulism), *C. perfringens* (gangrene and food poisoning), as well as the intestinal bug *C. difficile*, often called *C. diff* (severe diarrhea is one characteristic symptom). Other common gut bacteria whose function is to break down the amino acids from proteins are *Bacteroides*, *Propionibacterium*, *Streptococcus*, *Bacillus*, and *Staphylococcus*. Unchecked, these species of bacteria commonly overgrow when intestinal conditions favor protein fermentation—that is, when protein exceeds fiber consumption.

Competition for space and resources in the human gut can literally be a fight to the death. *Clostridia* has a particularly nasty trick that gives it an advantage. *Clostridia*, in essence, employs poison to eliminate its rivals. Its defense works this way: when *Clostridia* metabolizes protein, it secretes enzymes that aid in the fermentation of the amino acids tryptophan, phenylalanine, and tyrosine. While fermentation of these amino acids is not the preferred energy source for *Clostridia*, it relies on these macronutrients when other nutrients, namely fiber, are limited or not available. This process produces the *phenol* class of compounds as a waste product, which is toxic to other bacteria but not to *Clostridia*.[21] Since other cells (including human) have no metabolic use for phenols, the result is a toxic buildup of phenolic compounds in the large and small intestine. This metabolic pathway—from amino acid to phenol—is not playing nice in the playground. Phenol is a dead-end metabolite that provides no trophic feeding or synergistic relationship with other microbial or human cells. This chemical onslaught is *Clostridia*'s survival mechanism, in which it grabs an available nutrient and produces a toxin to ward off competition from other bacteria, because preferred nutrients—particularly fiber—are in short supply.

The consequences of phenolic overload to humans can also be severe. When phenols are detected by the host (again, us), it induces a stress response in the cells of the intestinal mucosa, resulting in inflammation, activation of glial cells, and increased glutamate signaling[22]— effects that are adverse to human health. A cascade of similar events, all leading to dysregulated glutamate signaling, is believed to be the mechanism underlying various types of cancers, including colon cancer.[23] This is an example of how a microbe induces an inflammatory response that increases glutamate release from our own cells. Our own cells increase glutamate production in order to sound the warning bells that things are not well.

To be clear, not all varieties of *Clostridia* present in our guts are bad actors in the human microbiome ecosystem. In fact, studies show that the presence of some *Clostridia* species may be critical for healthy brain function.[24] Critical neurotransmitters such as serotonin (mood and social behavior, digestion, sleep), glutamate (learning, memory, sensory signaling), GABA (gamma-aminobutyric acid, which has a calming effect), dopamine (reward-motivated behavior), norepinephrine (emotional regulation and learning), and hydrogen sulfide (signaling) are all examples of neurotransmitters produced from amino acid metabolism of microbes. So, to be fair, when naming names, it's a rare bacterium that is all good or all bad. When it comes to microbiome health, the critical features are balance and diversity.

Your Relationship with an Intimate Partner: Your Microbiome

If Jane Austen fans will forgive my paraphrasing her inimitable introduction to *Pride and Prejudice*, let me say that it is a truth universally acknowledged that bad relationships suck the energy out of you. Here I am talking about your relationship with your gut microbiome—probably the most intimate biological partnership we as humans experience after the umbilical cord is snipped.

So far you have read about how the microscopic denizens of our digestive tract aid digestion, manufacture critical vitamins and neurotransmitters, support our immune system, and help defend against disease-carrying invaders. We love them, right? But this relationship can go south, and at these times we may see our gut microbiota as soulless opportunists, fighting for turf and resources no matter what the cost to us (the host). After all, a seriously out-of-whack gut ecosystem can land us in the hospital and even turn deadly.

Our health depends on a healthy relationship with these trillions of microbes, and here I am going to explain briefly what many scientists think that relationship looks like—and how I think we can do better. A healthy relationship with our microbiota is often referred to as a *commensal* one—that is, one in which the microbe benefits and no harm is done to the human host. Some still mistakenly use this term as the optimal role. But we can do better than having a relationship that simply does no harm. Microbes eat our food, and we give them a place to live. Something that extracts energy from us should benefit us. Here are three basic types of relationships we can have with our microbes.

1. For health, we want a *mutual* relationship with our microbes, in which the microbes provide critical functions promoting human wellness and the human body provides nutrients that support the health of a diverse, abundant ecosystem.
2. A *commensal* relationship is one where the microbes don't harm the host but do not provide benefits to the host, who is providing benefits to the microbes—that is, we are being used. This health state is surviving, not thriving.
3. A *parasitic* relationship is a pathogenic or deleterious one, in which microorganisms are harming human health. Microbes are opportunistic and, when given the chance, their abundant growth can turn even a mutualistic relationship with a host into a pathogenic or parasitic one, often resulting in immune and inflammatory responses. And there are microbes that are harmful to the host, even in low numbers.

When we consider the metabolic cost of playing host to the wrong microbial partners, my point that a bad human–microbiome relationship will drain you of energy is literally true. The microbes in your gut create a chemical milieu that we must necessarily respond to. If the human cells in the intestinal mucosa are fighting the buildup of toxins in the digestive tract, are not getting the nutrients or essential metabolites that a well-balanced microbiome ecosystem provides, are combatting inflammation, and are being overwhelmed by excitatory glutamate signaling, there is no energy left for growth or wellness.

Communication

Another trope: good relationships are built on communication. Our gut talks to the brain and our brain talks to the gut. This is done through chemical signaling, and although we may not be consciously aware of this two-way conversation, we feel it.

One way in which microbes communicate with human cells is through the production of neurotransmitters, like serotonin, GABA, dopamine, norepinephrine, adrenaline, hydrogen sulfide, nitric oxide and, yes, of course, glutamate. These neurotransmitters affect our mood, not because Johnny Microbe wants us to be depressed and therefore releases glutamate, but because the production of glutamate serves the survival of Johnny Microbe. And when Johnny Microbe invites a bunch of friends who all are thriving on making and using glutamate, the human host feels an imbalance in the glutamate signaling. You don't feel *well*. The production of neurotransmitters from our microbial inhabitants is at the root of the research aimed at understanding the "gut–brain axis"—which has also given scientific insight into the term "gut feeling."

One thing science tells us is that changes in the numbers and types of microbes living in our guts influence glutamate signaling in our brains.[25] This is supported by research with mice,[26] in which changes in the level of brain glutamate were measured and correlated with changes in gut microflora. This finding is actually quite remarkable. Glutamate, a molecule that is found in every living thing, is the most primitive, evolutionarily conserved chemical messenger on the planet. It crosses the language barrier between us and bacteria and archaea, organisms so different that they are separated by billions of years of evolution. Glutamate is like a universal Morse code that allows the microbes within our gut to pass messages among themselves, and to us. Human glial cells are frequently the agents that sense glutamate produced by bacteria and initiate the body's response.

When considering our diet, we need to consider how our foods influence the conversation between us and our microbial partners. What we eat affects microbial metabolism, which in turn influences the glutamate load in the gut, which affects the brain. Don't be fooled: the communication goes both ways. Food cravings are one way microbes in our gut put in their demands for foods that promote their growth, often at the expense of human health.[27] The most studied example of food and addiction are obesity studies, where the particular microbial composition of obese individuals was shown to alter the dopamine reward system through gut–brain signaling. One result was suppressing participants' feeling of being "satisfied," causing people to overeat.

And what about mood? Here's a question to all: rather than treating depression with glutamate blocker drugs like ketamine, riluzole, and acamprosate, why not first determine how much mood dysfunction is being influenced by diet, and the effect of diet on gut microbial activity? While many of us ignore the association of our mood with our foods and gut microbial activity, the science continues to support the connection.[28]

The bottom line is, we want to have a mutual relationship with our microbes in which we provide benefits to them and they provide benefits to us. There is much we can eat to make that happen. The greatest impact on our relationship with our microflora is the 50 tons of food we choose to eat over a lifetime.

Microbe Migration

What would you do if your home was toxic or there was no food? You would move. This is the survival choice for the trillions of organisms in the colon when their human host eats an imbalanced diet. When too few nutrients reach the large intestine, microbial communities that normally reside there move up the GI tract to the small intestine, searching for available nutrients. In the small intestine, these microbes are forced to compete with each other, compete with microorganisms already established in the small intestine, and do all this in a section of the GI tract much different than what they are accustomed to.

This migration is not a formula for wellness. Populations of microorganisms that don't compete successfully die, leading to a lack of diversity and new opportunities for overgrowth of fewer species. That's not good for human cells, either. Our human microbiome ecosystem evolved with microbial populations occupying specific niches within our digestive tracts, and a mutually beneficial relationship with our microbiota depends on fermentation taking place in these specific locations. If this doesn't happen, human cells (which can't pick up and move to a different region of body when the nutrients go away) are left malnourished or, at worst, awash in toxins created by microbes adjusting to their new environment and new roles.

Translocation of gut microbes is the biggest migration problem facing our health. Let's look at an example of a common consequence of overgrowth in the small intestine and a diet high in processed foods, particularly refined carbohydrates, that feeds a newly relocated microbial population. This subject deserves special mention because this microbial imbalance in the small intestine (described earlier with regard to SIBO) is occurring in epidemic proportions. The particular example I dive into next has to do with alcohol.

Intestinal Production of Alcohol

Modern societies have a greater addiction to alcohol than we realize. As a part of my interest in how various foods impact health, I started examining blood and urine metabolites of various ill populations. I looked mainly at chronic fatigue and cardiovascular disease in adults, and autism, sensory dysregulation, and ADHD in pediatric groups, but I also analyzed an assortment of inflammatory/neuroinflammatory conditions such as migraines and diabetes. In both adult and pediatric populations, GI symptoms often accompanied their other symptoms. In pediatric autism groups, the prevalence of GI symptoms is 75 percent. I, too, observed many GI symptoms in my daughter before we started eating differently.

Some of the many symptoms reported in these patient populations included bloating soon after eating meals, constipation, abdomen pain, brain fog after eating (I used to call it a food coma), headaches, strong cravings for simple carbohydrates or sugars, waking up in middle of night and unable to fall back to sleep, imbalanced energy (excess fatigue or hyperactivity), and bouts of irritability, lack of coordination, or giddiness. What I discovered to be a common theme in these cases was the overproduction of various types of alcohols from the fermentation of simple carbohydrates and sugars in the small intestine, which I was able to observe in lab results. Yes, intoxication from alcohol that your own body produces is a thing—this disorder is called auto-brewery syndrome or gut fermentation syndrome, and a full-blown case of it can get you arrested for drunk driving, even if you haven't had a drop to drink.[29]

Not many parents will connect the dots that their young child may be drunk and becoming addicted to alcohol from the fermentation of simple sugars and carbohydrates in the small intestine. But when you think about it, many fungal and bacterial groups ferment sugar to alcohol. Take vodka, for example, which is produced from the fermentation of potatoes by yeast. This is how we make commercial alcohol, after all. We all produce some alcohol as part of microbial fermentation in the GI tract, and it is readily absorbed by our bodies. However, excess alcohol production can start to drastically alter human cell metabolism, depending on the amount of alcohol and time of exposure. I posit that what is often referred to as non-alcoholic liver disease may actually be caused by unintentional alcohol exposure due to alcohol production from microbial fermentation in the gut. Alarmingly, this type of liver disease is increasing in children in modern societies.

This doesn't happen all at once. Before the liver is impacted, chronic exposure to alcohol changes cell function, starting with epithelial cells (the innermost lining of intestine) and immune cells in the gastrointestinal tract. Rather than metabolizing sugars, the human cell metabolizes the alcohol, which is toxic and needs to be eliminated. The energy and enzymes necessary to metabolize alcohol cause a significant impairment in glucose (sugar) metabolism and the cell goes into lipogenesis (fat-producing) mode—thus the reason prolonged alcohol exposure increases fats in the liver. Symptoms from prolonged alcohol exposure often include acetone breath, which is caused by excess ketone production. These metabolic changes are also common in cirrhosis of the liver, diabetes, and alcoholic syndrome. Non-alcoholic liver disease in adults and children is likely the same mechanism as alcoholic liver disease.

Few people will look at seven-year-olds and suspect their behavioral problems and moods are due to alcohol addiction, but modern diets may be creating more pediatric alcoholics than we realize. To learn more about this process and symptoms to look out for, see chapter 7, "Glutamate and Disease."

One of the consequences of alcohol metabolism in our cells is the increased production of glutamate, which is part of the reward mechanism leading to alcohol addiction. Like so many of our reward systems, addiction to alcohol is neurologically wired through glutamate signaling. You will find more on addiction related to glutamate signaling in chapter 7.

Alcohol toxicity from imbalanced microbial metabolism is just one example of the many unintended consequences that come from fermentation of food within our GI tract. While there may be various causes that result in microbial imbalance (antibiotics, infection, or trauma, for example), one factor will continue to feed this imbalance: a poorly balanced diet. Unfortunately, the phenomenon of microbes creating a toxic-waste site in our gut is not only possible, it is common in the modern diet.

Our human metabolism, and our genes, cannot adapt easily to the shifting migration of billions or trillions of microbes and their associated metabolites, which are important to *our* metabolic, immunologic, and neurologic functions. The solution to the migration issue is straightforward: provide our microbiome with a hospitable environment in the proper place in the digestive tract through balanced ratios of nutrients in foods. That is the topic for chapter 8, "Roadmap to Health: The REID Food Lifestyle." But before we go there, let's connect the dots linking glutamate in the diet with inflammation. Chronic inflammatory diseases are the leading cause of death in modern societies. For that reason alone, it's important to understand how what America eats is fueling the crisis. That is the topic of chapter 6, "The Slow-Growing Fire: Inflammation and Diet." Following that, we will learn how glutamate signaling may be connected to myriad specific diseases in chapter 7. If you need any more motivation for considering the REID lifestyle, that is the chapter you must read.

6

The Slow-Growing Fire

INFLAMMATION AND DIET

WHAT LED ME TO INVESTIGATE THE ROLE OF DIET IN INFLAMMATION was a physician at the Lucile Packard Children's Hospital observing that Taylor's EEG brain scan, during the height of her autism symptoms, showed evidence of brain inflammation—or in medical parlance, "encephalitis and general encephalopathy." From college immunology classes, I had a basic understanding of what inflammation was. I resolved to learn more about brain inflammation and find the connection between it and my daughter's symptoms. I soon learned that inflammation of the brain usually is a sign that there is inflammation elsewhere, or even throughout the whole body.

Inflammation is one weapon in an arsenal of biological weapons that protects the body from things that would do us harm. Bad actors like pathogens (e.g., viruses and harmful bacteria), toxins (e.g., snake venom and poison ivy), and injuries (e.g., twisted ankle and cut finger) all elicit an inflammatory response. This is great if the battle against harmful agents is won quickly, but inflammation is energetically exhausting and takes its toll on the body when it persists. In Taylor's case, a chronically inflamed brain meant that there was little energy left over for learning, relating to us, and managing emotions.

Chronic inflammation is a harbinger of disease, and reducing inflammation is the goal of a large number of drugs and therapies targeting a great many conditions. Reducing inflammation is one of the goals of the REID food lifestyle—inflammation is the "I" in REID. As you will learn, glutamate and inflammation go hand in hand, and efforts to manage inflammation are made more difficult when your food is inducing a chronic excitatory and/or inflammatory response in your body.

A Quick Course in Inflammation

Anyone who has had an injury or infection will recognize the four signs of inflammation: redness, heat, swelling, and pain. For example, if you burn your finger, your reaction is immediate pain, which tells the body that cells are being injured and initiates an *immune response*. Immune system cells release inflammatory signals that cause small blood vessels to dilate, bringing more blood and more immune system cells to the site of the injured tissue. More immune cells promote healing, but the influx of more blood also makes the injured tissue red and hot. In addition, protein-rich fluid seeps out of the dilated blood vessels and into tissues to help the injured tissue. This causes swelling. The increased volume of fluid in inflamed tissues also presses against nerve endings, and the result is you feel more pain.

Glutamate is one of a cast of characters that mediates inflammation, and a defining characteristic of inflammation is increased levels of glutamate at the site of inflammation.[1] The higher the glutamate level, the more severe the inflammatory response.[2] Because glutamate is an excitatory neurotransmitter, it communicates different degrees of "ouch," depending on the severity of inflammation. Like redness, heat, and swelling, pain has a protective function, too. If something hurts, you tend to shield or favor it, thus keeping the affected body part safe from further injury.

Inflammation and the accompanying redness, heat, swelling, and pain are designed to help heal. Chronic inflammation, however, leads to disease. Diseases associated with inflammation of specific tissues are so common that they have their own names, ending with *itis*. Arthritis, colitis, bronchitis, appendicitis, tonsillitis, encephalitis, cystitis . . . you get the picture.

The fact is, chronic inflammatory diseases are the leading cause of death in modern societies. Cardiovascular disease, cancer, respiratory disease—mechanistically, the pathologies of these diseases are often indistinct from each other, with the common mechanism being chronic inflammation. I'll describe how inflammation and glutamate relate to specific diseases in more detail in chapter 7, "Glutamate and Disease," but for now we will connect the dots between glutamate and inflammation and look at the long-term consequences of inflammation on the body.

A Bucket of Inflammation

Modern diets and environments contain so many potentially inflammatory agents that many of us walk around in a state of chronic inflammation. When the immune system is responding to too many immune activators, the inflammation load is high and our "inflammation bucket" can reach a tipping point.

Think of your inflammation bucket as the sum total of all the inflammation signaling occurring at any time in your body. And there is *always* some inflammation signaling occurring. Even at our healthiest, the activities of daily living (ADL) bring us in contact with infectious agents (think germy doorknobs and keyboards). ADL subject us to myriad tiny injuries (think shaving or stubbing a toe). Simply moving through the day causes our bodies to be in a constant state of repair and restoration. All of this is normal.

A healthy immune and inflammatory system allows us to manage our ADL. What's not healthy is when our inflammation bucket is so full that normal ADL overflow the bucket, so to speak. Our immune system was not designed to manage an excessively high inflammatory load day in and day out. And for many in modern societies, there are far too many inflammation triggers, from physical injury to infectious agents to our food choices. Even the routine business of a cell becoming stressed can generate an inflammatory signal, sounding the alarm in the same way that a burn would. Cellular stress can take the form of a metabolic imbalance, such as glucose deprivation, or can be caused by exposure to toxins, such as daily consumption of alcohol. All this adds more inflammation chemicals to the inflammation bucket.

There is no one-size-fits-all measurement for a person's capacity to tolerate inflammation. Each person has their own uniquely sized inflammation bucket, established over a lifetime. Our inflammatory bucket begins to be defined with the genes (both human and microbiome) that are expressed as we develop, some even before birth. This inflammatory bucket continues to evolve through infancy and adulthood as our immune system matures and responds to our world. The best way to keep the inflammation bucket from spilling over is to reduce your exposure to inflammatory agents. Makes sense, doesn't it?

Consequences of Chronic Inflammation and Glutamate Signaling

One type of cell that connects glutamate signaling to the inflammatory pathway is the *glial cell*. Glial cells merit special mention because they have an outsized role in glutamate signaling. The primary job of glial cells is to protect neurons, but they also train neurons to be better attuned to the environment. How do glial cells do that? Glial cells mop up excess glutamate present in the extracellular space (see figure 4.1). This protects neurons from excessive random firing. When neural firing is needed, however, glial cells release proinflammatory signals like glutamate and other substances called *cytokines* to activate neurons.[3] Cytokines prime neurons to respond vigorously to certain environmental stimuli. With repeated exposure to the stimuli, these vigorous responses become imprinted on our neural network—this is the "training" I referred to when I said that glial cells train neurons to better respond to their environment. This works as it should—until our inflammation bucket is full. After that, relatively insignificant, non-noxious stimuli can overwhelm the system, resulting in chronic activation of the glial cells. At that point, glial cells no longer mop up glutamate but instead release it, and the spillover that ensues excites all neurons in its path.

When glial cells are chronically activated, chronic inflammation occurs. The all-too-common, damaging consequences of chronic inflammation are chronic pain, erosion of the body's protective barriers, and cancer. I'll talk about these consequences next, in that order.

Chronic Pain

All of us can relate to acute pain, and many of us experience chronic pain, particularly as we age. The purpose of acute pain is to alert us to situations that can do us harm. Pain fires up our nerve endings via glutamate signaling and sends a message to the brain: "That hurts. Stop doing that."[4]

Chronic pain is different. The pain signal does not shut off, and nothing you do, or stop doing, makes the pain go away. The consequences are debilitating.

If we think of chronic pain in the context of inflammation, we see that chronic pain occurs when a person's body senses a threat to the survival of cells, a threat that is constant and unrelenting. This causes the body's inflammatory pathways to be chronically activated. This chronic, elevated level of inflammation can cause a person's inflammation bucket to overflow with the slightest increase of their inflammatory load. Think of it this way: if your inflammation bucket is at full capacity, then the smallest inflammatory challenge—even one seemingly unrelated to chronic pain, such as consuming a bag of processed snack food—can provoke a reaction way out of proportion to the stimulus. Pain intensifies because your inflamed body simply can't handle any more inflammatory triggers.

Cruelly, the body's inability to calm down the nerve cells and dampen the inflammatory signal causes the number of glutamate receptors in cell membranes to actually *increase*, as cells gear up to accommodate the perceived threat. In this state, one becomes even more vulnerable and sensitive to glutamate signaling, and the result is more pain and swelling. The take-home message: the more inflamed an individual, the more sensitive the neurons are to glutamate. This is where diet becomes critical: research shows that glutamate in food increases inflammation.[5] If you are already inflamed, dietary glutamate could just push you over the edge.

Is there scientific evidence that diet contributes to emotional and physical pain? Yes.[6] Headaches, stomachaches, depression, anxiety, obsession … all of these conditions can be connected to MSG in the diet and imbalances in glutamate signaling.[7] There isn't much difference in the underlying mechanism between chronic emotional and physical pain, and often both symptoms are experienced in an individual simultaneously.[8] Many people don't know why they are getting frequent headaches or would think to attribute their feelings of depression to what they ate.[9] Yet the brain is aware of the level of inflammation in the gut and reacts accordingly. Not understanding the reason why they are feeling the way they do, people ignore the potential triggers and the inflammation bucket becomes more and more full.

Erosion of Protective Barriers

The body maintains an array of barriers, both microscopic and macroscopic, that have the important role of keeping things apart. For now, let's just say these barriers separate things that should be "inside" from things that need to be kept "outside." At the level of our cells, the thin cell membrane functions as this kind of barrier. Cells are constantly sensing the environment to determine what stays inside the cell, what should be kept out, and what is allowed to pass in and out across the cell membrane. Glutamate is one of the chemical messengers that allows cells to make these decisions by providing information on conditions on both sides of the barrier.

Chronic inflammation harms protective barriers by making them permeable, or "leaky." Below I give some examples of what that looks like. Let's start with the skin, and then dive into the body's increasingly smaller barriers and see how this is tied to glutamate.

Skin

We see our skin every day and are likely to be very aware of the visible signs of inflammation: a rash, eczema, skin eruptions, infection, or physical injury. Skin is the largest organ in the body and is often the first responder to environmental insults such as heat or cold, pollutants in the air, toxins in the water we bathe in, and ingredients in the products we apply to our bodies.

To understand what happens when the skin's protective barriers start to fail, you need to know that human skin consists of sheets of cells layered one on top of the other. The movement of substances between these layers is possible through highly regulated channels or pores between the cells called *tight junctions*. Tight junctions open or close to allow water and ions to pass. Intuitively, you can see how the integrity of tight junctions is essential for the skin to work as a barrier. Walls can't be effective if the gates are wide open.

The opening and closing of tight junctions are coordinated by a vast, weblike *glutamatergic* neural network that exists between the layers of skin. (Note that glutamatergic simply means "related to glutamate"; it is a term you see a lot if you are reading about this topic online.) The healthy functioning of this neural network is important because skin makes possible our sense of touch, the body's response to hydration and temperature, the regeneration of new skin after a wound, activation of inflammation, and our reaction to pain.[10] But what is happening with chronic skin inflammation, the hallmark of painful conditions like psoriasis? Or chronic skin infections like acne or fungus, and even more severe conditions, like skin cancer?

Chronically inflamed skin is a sign that the skin's glutamatergic network is out of kilter. The once highly orchestrated opening and closing of tight junctions becomes chaotic and, bit by bit, tight cell junctions become disorganized and loose. In this state, the gates open, and skin layers become more permeable to microbes and toxins. In chronic skin inflammatory conditions like psoriasis, the layers of skin no longer look like barriers. The layers let through the noxious agents our skin is meant to protect against.

Unfortunately, skin is also now more sensitive to stimuli that previously it could ignore. Even food can initiate an inflammatory response in the skin. Reacting to something you ate, you may experience an outbreak of hives, flushing of the face, or itching. Your skin is sending a signal, alerting you that your internal inflammatory load is becoming critically high.

Intestinal Wall

The intestinal wall is a protective lining that keeps undigested food and toxins in the intestines from entering the tissues of the body. Like skin, this gastrointestinal barrier consists of layers of cells joined together by tight junctions. Traffic across these layers is well controlled, with specific mechanisms that transport, digest, and absorb nutrients. And because humans can't be trusted about what they put in their mouths, the intestinal barrier has multiple strategies to protect us from the non-food items and pathogens we might ingest. To this end, the intestinal wall produces mucus and immune system antibodies.

A robust gastrointestinal tract is absolutely critical to wellness, and its healthy functioning is orchestrated by the largest assembly of neurons and glial cells existing outside the central nervous system. Aptly dubbed our "second brain," the enteric nervous system (ENS)[11] is a neural network that extends into the lining of the esophagus, stomach, small intestine, and colon. Our conscious awareness of what is going on in our gut is made possible by the vagus nerve, one of various nerves connecting the ENS in our abdomen with our brains. As you might expect by now, the two-way messaging between gut and brain is made possible by glutamate signalling. The gut feeling that this book and others talk about is literally the consequence of the many glutamate receptors that map all along the gastrointestinal tract from tongue to anus.[12] You can think of these sensors as a kind of taste receptor, cellularly the same as those in taste buds. These receptors are not associated with a flavor per se (like sour or sweet), but they do signal to the brain the same feeling of pleasure that our taste buds do—ergo, a gut feeling.

So how are glutamate and inflammation intertwined in the gastrointestinal tract? This brings us back to the role of glial cells.

Under homeostasis (business-as-usual, non-stress conditions), glial cells in the intestinal lining regulate digestion, motility (the muscle contractions that move digested food toward the anus), inflammation, immune responses, and are tasked with maintaining the integrity of the intestinal barrier.[13] Recall also that glial cells mop up excess glutamate as a way to protect neurons from abnormal signaling. However, when there is too much glutamate around and glial cells exhaust their capacity to take up any more, glial cells will *release* glutamate and activate neuronal signaling in the gut.[14] This is a little like an overly protective queen bee sensing a threat to her hive. When things really get bad, the queen bee (glial cell) sends out a chemical stress signal that rallies the worker bees (nearby neurons), sending them out of the hive, stinging and creating chaos and pain.

Now serious problems ensue (not with the bees but with the glial cells). In the presence of high levels of glutamate (stress conditions), glial cells change their physical shape and their function. They also increase the number of glutamate receptors on their cell membranes, which exacerbates inflammation and physical pain.[15] After prolonged exposure to glutamate, the physical changes in the glial cells start to increase the permeability—the leakiness—of the intestinal barrier. Further cell damage and cell death then occurs, resulting in more intestinal wall damage.[16]

The destruction or injury to glial cells and the resulting increase in intestinal permeability leads to many illnesses, including inflammatory bowel disease, necrotizing enterocolitis (a dangerous type of gut inflammation that can lead to holes forming in the wall of the intestine), irritable bowel syndrome, diabetes, autoimmune diseases, viral infections of nerve cells in the gut, and constipation.[17] The relationship is pretty straightforward: the degree of inflammation and the severity of diseases of the gut is correlated with the degree of intestinal permeability.[18]

The geeky scientist in me thinks this is amazing, and you might be asking yourself at this point: Does glutamate in *food* cause problems with intestinal wall permeability? Research says yes. We know that glutamate in food activates the vagus nerve (which I described earlier as linking the brain in your head with your "second brain" in your gut). Excessive firing of the vagus nerve leads to chronic activation of the "gut brain," which in turn leads to inflammation and intestinal disorders.[19]

Here are the details, for any readers who wish to evaluate the evidence for themselves: in humans, a dietary study demonstrated that most of the subjects who had irritable bowel syndrome (IBS) improved with eliminating MSG from their diet, and their IBS symptoms returned when MSG was added back.[20] In a study using dogs, dietary glutamate caused vagus nerve activation, which resulted in abnormal secretion of digestive enzymes,[21] which impacts digestion and can reduce absorption of nutrients. Wall erosion in the large intestine has been linked to MSG consumption in pigs, the animal model that most resembles the human GI tract. In this study, MSG consumption was associated with decreased amounts of tight junction protein in the large intestine.[22] Just like we saw in skin, tight junctions—and tight junction proteins—are critical to the integrity of the intestinal barrier. The same study also showed that MSG consumption results in a shift in microbial populations that secrete proinflammatory cytokines and toxins known to increase intestinal permeability. So yes, the scientific data show that dietary glutamate causes problems with intestinal wall permeability.

Blood-Brain Barrier (BBB)

You may recall the term "blood-brain barrier," introduced in chapter 4. The blood-brain barrier (BBB) can be described as a skin of semipermeable tissue that wraps the brain and keeps bad things, like pathogens and toxins, from leaking out of the bloodstream and entering the brain. What you might not know is that glutamate is one of the substances that generally stops at the blood-brain barrier, and for whom entry into and out of the brain is highly regulated.[23]

The reason for this is related to the critical role of glutamate in nerve conduction. Consider that the average human brain has about 86 billion neurons. These cells contain the highest concentration of glutamate of any cell in the body, concentrations that are an astonishing 5,000 to 20,000 times higher than that found in the surrounding extracellular fluid (see chapter 4). Remember, glutamate is an excitotoxin, and concentration of glutamate in the fluid outside brain cells must be kept low in order to keep our brain cells from misfiring. Blood can have glutamate concentrations a hundredfold higher than the fluid bathing the brain, which would be dangerous if somehow glutamate leaked from blood vessels into the brain. Why doesn't this happen? Scientists have always pointed to the blood-brain barrier, which has a well-tuned transport system for controlling the flow of glutamate to and from the brain. In healthy individuals, this works just fine. What has become clear, however, is that if glutamate signaling gets too high in the brain[24] or in blood, it causes inflammation and physical changes in the blood-brain barrier, making it more permeable to glutamate and other potential toxins.[25] As the blood-brain barrier becomes leaky, its protective function is compromised.

Numerous studies have shown that a permeable BBB exposes brain cells to the higher levels of free glutamate that naturally course through your blood vessels, leading to an excitotoxic effect[26] impacting brain cell metabolism and neural firing. More problematic, a harmful feedback loop can be established,[27] in which an initially slight metabolic dysfunction in brain cells increases permeability in the blood-brain barrier, which then allows glutamate and other substances to pass, which in turn amplifies the metabolic dysfunction of the brain cells.

My question to you, the reader, is this: if you could control your level of brain inflammation by diet, why wouldn't you? Unfortunately, traumas like brain injury, stroke, tumor, and some types of infection that result in chronic inflammation and long-term blood-brain barrier dysfunction[28] are difficult to remedy, but food choices can reduce progression of these conditions. There are other factors you can control, as well. You may not realize that *temporary* BBB permeability can occur as a result of stresses like sleep deprivation, infection, and glucose deprivation.[29] So here's some advice: eat right and get your sleep if you want to think right and feel right!

Cell Membrane

In this last example of how inflammation erodes your body's barriers, we drill down to the level of the cell. Here, the permeable barrier we are talking about is the *cell membrane*. The cell membrane encloses the cell and defines what is inside and outside. However, the cell membrane is more than a passive bag holding together the cell contents. The cell membrane takes an active role in facilitating the flow of nutrients and ions in and out of the cell. It protects the cell from environmental threats, and transmits and receives chemical signals to and from other cells. All these functions become compromised in the presence of excess glutamate, and the ensuing inflammation can result in damaged cell membranes and lead to cell death, or worse. What's worse than cell death? Read on.

Brain cells are good choices for examining these events. Because of the extraordinarily high concentration of glutamate inside brain cells, spring a leak in a brain cell membrane and a lot of excitatory glutamate can spill into the space between brain cells.

Recall that the inflammatory response is primarily a defense mechanism, designed to keep us healthy. At the cellular level, however, we can see the downside of the protective inflammatory response. For example, if there is a physical injury to the brain that damages cells, the flood of glutamate that leaks from the damaged cells, and the increased glutamate signaling that occurs as excited glial cells try to rescue the injured neurons, can become a very serious threat to our well-being. A cascade of toxicity can ensue—a "glutamate storm"—in which a dangerous amount of glutamate leaks out of brain cells into the extracellular fluid. This in turn alters the function and metabolism of nearby cells, causing *them* to leak glutamate. In the classic progression of inflammation, the excitatory response can be exported to other regions of the brain as glutamate signaling involves more and more nerve cells. The inflammatory chain reaction can cause long-term damage or can turn deadly if not managed quickly. And there is another cost: the inflammatory response is energetically expensive and requires a lot of calories. This means that an inflamed brain is an exhausted brain, with little energy left to support the activities of daily living.

All that said, the take-home message is simple: glutamate is a chemical essential for maintaining healthy barriers all throughout the body, and it must be kept in balance for optimal health.[30] Elevated concentrations of glutamate, whether from diet or an adverse life event, leads to inflammation and, when left unchecked, results in the erosion of critically important protective barriers.

Cancer

What's worse than cell death? You have just read how inflammation erodes precious protective barriers and alters the functioning of a cell, sometimes to the point that the cell dies. We can recover from thousands of cells dying this way, but when cells don't die and instead make changes that allow them to survive in an unhealthy, inflammatory environment, we can be faced with an outcome that may be worse than dead cells. What's worse than a dead cell is a cancerous cell. Cancer is another consequence of chronic inflammation and cellular metabolism gone awry.

We now know that many types of cancers are directly linked to excess glutamate. Excess glutamate signaling, the signature of chronic inflammation, is beneficial to the survival of cancer cells, and it can transform a healthy cell to a cancerous one. I'll describe how this happens in chapter 7, but the point is that in an inflamed body, glutamate signaling becomes an agent for initiating and promoting cancer.[31] As one group of researchers states,

> Aberrant glutamate signaling has been demonstrated to participate in the initiation and progression of a broad spectrum of cancers, including glioma, melanoma, breast cancer, and prostate cancer, suggesting the oncogenic functions of glutamate signaling in cancers.[32]

The critical words to me are "initiation and progression" of cancers. Aberrant glutamate signaling is not just a byproduct of cancer—it participates in the *initiation and progression* of cancer! In other words, aberrant glutamate signaling *causes* cancer (initiation) and *facilitates the growth* of cancer (progression)—many different kinds of cancer—and it does this by transforming cell metabolism, one cell at a time. This is eye-opening.

The main takeaway here is that inflammation, regardless of its root cause (infection, injury, dietary glutamate, inflammatory foods, stress, etc.) increases glutamate signaling, leading to diseases, even cancer. Chronic inflammation kills.

REID Food Lifestyle: Reduced Excitatory Inflammatory Diet

I am going to introduce the REID regimen with a story about Lyme disease. Certain pathogenic bacteria, such as the one associated with

Lyme disease (*Borrelia burgdorferi*), actually prefer glutamate-rich environments in their human hosts because they are unable to make this amino acid themselves. In fact, once *Borrelia burgdorferi* infects a person through the bite of a deer tick, it enters the bloodstream and actively seeks locations in the body where glutamate concentrations are the highest, usually areas where there is inflammation.[33] There, the Lyme disease pathogen finds readily available what it needs to maximize its virulence and wreak havoc on its human host.[34] Despite these bacteria being associated with humans throughout history, infection rates have increased in modern times. One has to wonder if the now-common prevalence of chronic inflammation in the human population has presented an opportunity for these organisms to become more pathogenic, and that is why more people are getting sick from Lyme disease.

Even if we're not keeping company with deer ticks, for many of us, the inflammation bucket is full and is easily tipped with our activities of daily living. Here's where diet becomes important, because food choices offer significant opportunities to lower inflammation. For many, foods choices are often what is tipping the bucket. Foods should nourish and help keep inflammatory events rare, not chronic. Glutamate is one ingredient in food that has a known role in activating the inflammatory and immune response.[35] But glutamate is not the only actor. There are many other ingredients in foods that induce inflammation, and subsequently can increase glutamate release from our own cells (human and microbial). Part of balancing glutamate metabolism is managing inflammation—and what inflames you may be very different than what inflames another person. This is true even within the same family, although genetics can and do play a role in inflammatory responses.

Here's one way I experienced the inflammation bucket before Taylor and I changed our food lifestyle to REID. Taylor and I had a number of environmental allergies. Taylor tested with high levels of the allergy antibody IgE to both cats and dust mites. Well, we had a cat, so we kept the cat out of Taylor's room and routinely vacuumed and dusted. If the cat came near Taylor, she experienced typical allergy symptoms, like runny nose and watery, itchy eyes. In my inflammation bucket, I had various pollen allergies throughout the year. For two months, twice a year, I felt like I had a long cold.

After we changed to REID, Taylor's allergies to cats and dust were significantly reduced. If she touched the cat and didn't wash her hands, she could still experience some allergy symptoms, but the upshot was that she could now touch the cat and even snuggle with our furry family member without consequence. The cat was in Taylor's room frequently, and the cat visiting her in other areas of the house no longer bothered her. This was very good news for the cat, and a sign of Taylor's increasing tolerance, consistent with a decrease in her overall inflammatory load.

As for me, I no longer experience the pollen allergies I had for 40 years. I can garden, ride my bike, and hike, and not experience the sudden onslaught of runny nose and sneezing fits that once invariably came with the seasons. Often when I tell people this story, their surprised response reflects the common belief that environmental allergies are part of an individual's bucket that can't be changed, and that environmental allergies have nothing to do with diet. But that's not true. Your individual sensitivity to the world is all about your overall inflammation load, and how a certain load produces certain symptoms in you, the individual.

The REID food lifestyle focuses on reducing inflammation from a variety of food sources. The foods in the REID lifestyle are generally good for everyone because of the benefit of reducing your inflammation bucket and balancing glutamate signaling. You can't balance glutamate signaling if you are inflamed. And proper nutrients are critical for restoring energy balance following an inflammatory response.

What I have learned in my own experience, and through working with many people along their food lifestyle journey, is that the following three routines top the list for helping lower one's inflammation load:

1. *Increase consumption of high-fiber, nutrient-rich vegetables.* We've been hearing about this routine for a long time, and it's an inevitable move to make once a person accepts all the research. Yes, I'll even discuss in the final chapter how to get a two-year-old

to consume more kale or dandelion greens. Change can happen, and healthy food is something worth fighting for. Also remember that the trillions of microbes that are in your GI tract also want fiber for their fuel. The byproducts from microbial fiber fermentation in the gut—bacterial metabolites—are enormously beneficial to human health.

2. *Remove ultraprocessed foods.* Commercial processing destroys fiber and the nutritional content of "real" foods. Sadly, there is little nutritional value in the majority of foods available in the supermarket. Worse, food processing incorporates various additives during manufacturing, such as glutamate, to make the food marketable. Commercially processed foods contain the majority of excitotoxic and inflammatory additives. Chapter 2, "Can't Eat Just One," provides a list of food ingredients you want to avoid.

3. *Remove refined sugars.* We evolved to use glucose from whole foods for energy, but in home kitchens today we can sweeten food using refined sugars from beets, coconut, agave, maple trees, and cane. In industrial kitchens, a staggering amount of refined sugar is added to processed foods, and these various sugars are in everything from mayonnaise to breakfast cereal. The consequences are serious. When our sugar level is too high, the body responds by trying to block excess glucose from entering our cells. Medically, this is called *insulin dysregulation*, and it leads to diabetes. Refined sugars are an easy fuel for our gut microbes, too. With a diet high in sugar, we create lazy microbes that ferment the glucose, have massive parties with ever-expanding colonies, and overgrow in the upper intestinal tract. The waste products from their carrying-on—alcohols and aldehydes—interfere with our own cells, producing a hangover-like state, just like we went to a party ourselves. More on diabetes in chapter 7.

These are the top three lifestyle changes that would go a long way toward reducing the inflammation bucket. There's more that can be done, but this is a good start. For the whole shebang, see chapter 8, "Roadmap to Health: The REID Food Lifestyle."

In summary, everyone can give their body a fighting chance to avoid chronic inflammation from foods by eliminating common inflammatory foods and adding plenty of foods that are known to reduce inflammation. However, there's an individual component to inflammation that makes each person's experience unique. The individual journey begins by becoming more aware of what other foods in your diet, specific to you, may be causing inflammation. A food sensitivity to sunflower seeds, for example, may create a problem for one individual, whereas sunflower seeds are a great protein, fat, fiber, and mineral source for most other people. Becoming more aware of your body's response to food is a huge part of the journey with REID.

We can start by looking at some of the disorders and diseases you may be experiencing or are susceptible to, which is the subject of the next chapter.

7

Glutamate and Disease

Do you know a kid who seems to exist on a diet of processed food, wanting only bags of snacks, chicken nuggets, and frozen pizza? You know this is unhealthy, but what you might not know is that the problem with processed food goes beyond its load of sugar, salt, and fat. Processed foods also contain excess glutamate (MSG), added by food manufactures to make the foods irresistible.

The effects of glutamate-laced processed foods can be profound, especially for individuals who already have an underlying disease that involves *glutamate dysregulation*. Expect to hear that term a lot. Glutamate dysregulation refers to any metabolic and/or neurological imbalance that ensues when glutamate—a neurotransmitter and metabolite essential for keeping our bodies working properly—is not adequately controlled.

In this chapter, I describe diseases that are directly linked to glutamate dysregulation. Addiction, ADHD, Alzheimer's disease, autism, cancer, multiple sclerosis, obesity, Parkinson's disease, schizophrenia . . . the list is long, and troubling. For most of these diseases, glutamate dysregulation is expressed as an imbalance in excitatory to inhibitory (E/I) signaling, a term describing whether a cell is activated (excited) or resting (inhibited).

Addiction

Perhaps the largest and most widespread impact of excessive glutamate signaling is the role of the glutamatergic system in addiction. At the time of writing this chapter, the grim truth is that more than 40 million Americans ages 12 and older have a substance abuse disorder involving opiates, alcohol, and/or other drugs.[1] In 2021, U.S. deaths from overdoses exceeded 100,000.[2] Addiction is a major emotional and financial cost to society, and addictions aren't limited to drugs and alcohol. What we are learning is that food and the use of electronic devices are also addicting. In modern societies, compulsive behaviors in these two areas now top the compulsive use charts. All of these addictions are neurologically wired through glutamate signaling. Yep, that's right, every single addiction is mapped onto our nervous system through the glutamate receptors on our nerve cells.

Addiction, when it becomes a health issue, is defined as maladaptive compulsive behaviors, often involving the consumption of a substance. In addition to drugs, the behavior can include compulsive ingestion of substances that we consider "good," and are even essential for survival, like food. The compulsive behavior can also involve obsessive and intrusive thoughts, and sex. As defined in the *Diagnostic and Statistical Manual of Mental Disorders* (DSM-V), compulsive-use disorder in individuals is characterized by preoccupation, escalation, tolerance, denial, and a series of medical, psychological, and social consequences directly related to the continuation of the behavior.[3]

Whatever the addiction is, it starts with a substance-induced or behavior-induced altered state that a person consciously experiences as pleasurable. On a molecular level, the substance or behavior either *lights up* the reward centers in the brain, releasing the "feel-good" neurotransmitter dopamine (as in the case of nicotine or amphetamines), or *inhibits* the neural circuitry with the release of a different neurotransmitter, the molecule gamma aminobutyric acid, or GABA (as in the case of alcohol and opiates). To the individual, either is a good thing. Depressed? Have a cigarette and get a boost. Anxious? A glass of wine—or two or three—will help you relax. All these functions—stimulation and sedation—are mediated by glutamate signaling. Over time, the repetition of the behavior causes a change in a person's glutamate receptor map.

The energy expended on reworking the glutamate receptor map is felt later, during daily life activities. In other words, when the high wears off, the depressed person feels a little more depressed than they did before, and the anxious person a little more anxious. To "feel normal" again, a person continues the compulsive behavior or substance use.

Decades of research point to glutamate dysregulation as the molecular mechanism underlying addiction.[4] The fact that glutamate regulates the release of dopamine is not well appreciated, but this turns out to be critical in understanding addiction and myriad other disorders, such as ADHD and Parkinson's disease, as we shall see.

While a comprehensive examination of the scientific literature on addiction is beyond the scope of this chapter, let's look at a few key studies.

Drug Use

Brain images of cocaine-addicted individuals show that using cocaine increases glutamate signaling. Take away the cocaine, and glutamate-mediated neural activity in the brain goes down. Researchers rank the severity of cocaine addiction by measuring how much glutamate signaling increases during exposure to the drug, and observing the length of time the signaling remains abnormal when the drug is taken away.[5] In one study, researchers examining chemical brain changes associated with methamphetamine addiction found that glutamate concentration in the brain was directly correlated with the duration of drug use—the longer one was using methamphetamine, the more glutamate in the brain.[6]

Alcohol Addiction

Consumption of alcoholic beverages is prevalent in the United States among adults and older children. The National Institute on Alcohol Abuse and Alcoholism reports that in 2018, 7.1 million young people ages 12 to 20 reported that they had drunk alcohol beyond "just a few sips" in the past month, and 861,000 reported binge drinking on five or more days over the previous month. In 2019, more than one in four adults ages 18 and older reported binge drinking within the past month.[7]

When the urge to drink becomes compulsive, drinking can lead to alcohol addiction. The neurological basis behind the numbing effect of alcohol and its miserable sidekicks, impaired cognitive function and increased pain tolerance, is attributed to reduced glutamate signaling in the brain. This reduction in brain activity (inhibitory signaling) is temporary, however. As the body metabolizes the ingested alcohol and it is eliminated, the suppression in glutamate signaling is followed by a rebound in brain activity as the body rebalances E/I signaling. This reset can sometimes be felt as a burst of energy or inability to sleep. The resulting excitatory (E) state can produce withdrawal symptoms such as agitation, anxiety, and disorientation, and result in cell damage.[8]

Chronic exposure to alcohol is accompanied by increased numbers of glutamate receptors on cell surfaces and, more important, changes in the *activity* of these receptors, which increase a person's tolerance to repeated alcohol exposure. More alcohol is then required to achieve intoxication.[9] In this way an alcoholic's glutamate map is redrawn as it adapts to chronic exposure to alcohol.

I want to point out that sometimes alcohol exposure is not a conscious choice. Such is the case when alcohol is produced during microbial fermentation of the food in one's gut. This can occur at any age and can even impact a developing fetus if a woman is pregnant. The neurological effects are particularly harmful for the unborn because of alcohol's ability to suppress glutamate signaling, which disrupts synapse development in the brain.[10] In children, who are busy learning about the world and are forming many new synapses, unintentional alcohol exposure can create challenges. Imagine, for example, how difficult it is for children to focus on schoolwork if they are tipsy.

One of my cases involved a seven-year-old boy I will call Henry, who exhibited disruptive behaviors in class. In addition to behavioral concerns, his parents reported digestive complaints such as bloating, constipation, and diarrhea. The boy was also always hungry and hyperactive, which suggested to me energy imbalance issues. My hunch about what was going on gained support when the parents showed me blood and urine panels indicating high levels of metabolites associated with bacteria and yeast, which can be a sign of small intestinal microbial overgrowth. In this case, there was also evidence that alcohol was involved in the boy's metabolic energy cycle. I asked about Henry's symptoms. Did he frequently act silly or laugh out of context? Did he have poor coordination, or did he have mood swings, quickly transitioning from elation to irritation or anger? The dad chimed in and said, "Yes! It's almost like he's acting like these drunk people I pick up off the streets at night." (Henry's father is a city police officer.) When I explained that I thought their son *was* drunk and explained how that could be, both parents were floored, and then relieved. This made sense and was something they could address by making changes to their son's diet. My food recommendations successfully and quickly resolved Henry's digestive and energy imbalance issues, allowing him to focus on school and engage in the important work of learning.

Post-Traumatic Stress Disorder

Why include post-traumatic stress disorder in a discussion about addiction? PTSD, characterized by reactive fight/flight responses, can neurologically resemble substance addiction. While no one *wants* to experience trauma or fear, the more our body experiences events that "trigger" fear or anger, the more our body becomes wired for it—wiring which, of course, is mediated by glutamate.[11] In fact, simply recalling a traumatic event and experiencing the feelings associated with it contributes to a *hyper*glutamatergic state that can neurologically resemble the experience of drug users. The cruel irony is that, while experiencing PTSD-triggering events is horrific, in the absence of these events the body experiences a *hypo*glutamatergic state—lower than normal glutamate signaling—which is also acutely distressful. Paradoxically, a person might try to relieve distress caused by the hypoglutamatergic state by actively seeking new stressful situations or engaging in substance abuse.[12]

I want to leave this section on a hopeful note. We know that compulsive-use disorders neurologically wire the brain, and glutamate signaling is the molecular mechanism underlying addiction behavior. This maladapted signaling is enabled because of the *plasticity of neurons*—the ability of the brain to adapt to its chemical environment, learn, and forge new pathways. This plasticity is also the solution. Overcoming addiction requires neurons to rewire the glutamate signaling pathways that support compulsive behaviors and replace them with new neural pathways. In fact, pharmaceutical companies have spent untold millions of dollars on glutamate blockers and other glutamate-related drug therapies with this very goal in mind. No one reading this book will be surprised to learn that I believe a healthy diet, free from added glutamate and processed food, is the first step to an addiction-free life.

Alzheimer's Disease

Alzheimer's disease is characterized by loss of memory and the presence of protein deposits in the brain called tangles and plaques. Approximately 50 million people worldwide are living with Alzheimer's or a related form of dementia. In the United States, an estimated 5.8 million adults of all ages have Alzheimer's. Of these, around 5.5 million are 65 years and older and approximately 300,000 are younger and have early onset Alzheimer's disease.[13]

As is true with many neurodegenerative diseases, Alzheimer's is typified by a loss of neurons. The mechanism believed to be responsible for the loss of neurons is excess glutamate signaling. Remarkably, this association with Alzheimer's was proposed nearly 30 years ago.[14] Thousands of studies later, the role of glutamate and overstimulated glutamate receptors remains the accepted central mechanism of the disease.[15]

How might this relate to plaques and tangles, the most visible signature of Alzheimer's disease in brain scans? These structures are comprised of two different proteins; plaques are made up of beta amyloid protein and tangles consist of a protein called tau. An increase in beta amyloid protein is directly linked to aberrant activity of a type of glutamate receptor called NMDA receptors. NMDA receptors also regulate the production of tau protein and determine whether this protein gets phosphorylated (chemically modified) in brain cells. The detail about phosphorylation is important, because it is the phosphorylated version of tau that is involved in the formation of tangles. If NMDA glutamate receptors are overstimulated, it creates an abundance of the phosphorylated tau protein—a hallmark in the pathology of Alzheimer's disease.[16]

Memantine is one of the first drugs approved for Alzheimer's for which the mechanism of action is to block glutamate from binding to NMDA glutamate receptors. Because of the numerous side effects, this drug has not proven to be as useful as was hoped. Yet the drug continues to be prescribed for other diseases, such as autism. This is just another example of the pharmaceutical industry offering drugs that block the action of glutamate, without addressing why glutamate receptors are being overstimulated in the first place. Alzheimer's is typically a late onset disease, and it is not a stretch to suggest that the excitotoxic effects of decades of exposure to the enormous amount of glutamate—MSG—that has entered the food supply could cause glutamate receptors to be chronically overstimulated, making one more vulnerable to Alzheimer's and related diseases.

Anxiety

Anxiety is the most common mood disorder diagnosed in the United States today, affecting more than 40 million adults. MSG consumption can often induce anxious behaviors, and evidence for this comes from the lab. In experiments with mice fed MSG, researchers observed erratic behaviors in mice navigating a maze, increased grooming, and a decrease in activities related to the rearing of offspring—behaviors classically associated with anxiety in these animals.[17] Although it is known that anxiety is associated with increased glutamate signaling in humans, approaches to manage the disorder don't examine diet but instead employ drugs to balance glutamate signaling.

Attention Deficit (Hyperactivity) Disorder (ADHD)

ADHD is characterized by persistent and developmentally inappropriate levels of overactivity, inattention, and impulsivity. According to the CDC, between 2016 and 2019, 13 percent of children between the ages of 12 and 17 years were diagnosed with ADHD.[18] Think about it. This means that in a typical classroom of 22 to 25 students, on average, two or three students will be diagnosed with ADHD. Put in these terms, you can see how the financial impact on school resources and programs is considerable.

Much of our insight into ADHD has come from studies focused on the dopamine reward system. In the brain, dopamine functions as the "feel good" neurotransmitter, signaling whether an outcome is desirable. This in turn influences whether a person is motivated to achieve that outcome. Some of the behaviors that define ADHD, such as poor motivation and lack of impulse control, are consistent with a weak dopamine reward system.

As I mentioned previously in connection with addiction, underappreciated in ADHD research is how dopamine's mode of action is dependent on other neurotransmitters, including glutamate.[19] Dopamine release is regulated by glutamate,[20] which suggests that if dopamine is not balanced, glutamate is likely involved. In fact, a study involving brain imaging of ADHD subjects showed increased levels of glutamate in the anterior cingulate cortex, a part of the brain thought to be responsible for impulse control, reward anticipation, decision making, and emotion.[21] How much glutamate was elevated corresponded to the ADHD subject's level of impulsivity and hyperactivity.

Diagnoses of ADHD and autism are often accompanied by some degree of auditory processing dysfunction, and this can be associated with glutamate signaling as well. It is known that glutamate excitotoxicity can damage the cochlea in the inner ear. The net effect of cochlear damage is to make sound, such as speech, less understandable, and it does this by decreasing the efficiency at which sound is translated into signals sent to the brain.[22] You can imagine how much more difficult it is to communicate with a child who can hear, but whose brain can't translate sound into meaningful words because of cochlear damage.

Other studies have demonstrated that glutamate injected into newborn rats is excitotoxic to the auditory system, producing high-frequency hearing loss.[23] This is further evidence of glutamate-mediated misfiring creating an excitatory/inhibitory (E/I) imbalance. In this case, a nervous system "out of sync" leads to auditory processing disorders.

I ask: if glutamate excitotoxicity is at the center of these behavioral and sensory disorders, why *wouldn't* a person try reducing one's environmental exposure to the large amount of glutamate present in the modern food supply? I point to a well-done, peer-reviewed dietary study that demonstrated the drastic improvements in symptoms of ADHD subjects brought about by changing diet.[24] In this study, participants consumed no processed foods and ate only whole foods. While the intent of this dietary study wasn't specifically to remove glutamate, ingesting only whole foods in effect eliminated added MSG and glutamate-enriched factory foods from the diet. This study was done in the Netherlands and Belgium, not the United States.

Autism

Autism spectrum disorder (ASD) is characterized by impaired social ability, poor communication skills, and repetitive behaviors. The percent of children afflicted with this devastating condition increases every year. Autism rates in 2000 were 1 in 150 children; by 2014 it was 1 in 59 children and in 2021, 1 in 44 children.[25]

At the time of this writing, there are no biomarkers, blood tests, or genetic traits for diagnosing autism. ASD is genetically and clinically varied. As its name indicates, autism spectrum disorder embraces a spectrum of clinical presentations. In recognition of this diversity, a common saying in the autism community is "once you've met a person with autism, you've met one person with autism."

Even within individuals, autism symptoms can be expressed idiosyncratically. For example, before we removed processed food and other sources of glutamate in her diet, my daughter Taylor exhibited extreme sensitivities to sounds, but only some sounds. She had this cute little stuffed animal, a cow, that when squeezed made a long "moo" sound. Once it started, the sound had to run its course and couldn't be shut off. One day I was on our outside deck and I accidentally stepped on the toy, causing the "moo" sound. Taylor immediately panicked. She covered her ears and ran in circles, trying to cope with the noise. I couldn't shut it off. To calm her, I chucked the cow over the deck, getting rid of the noise and the cow. Taylor immediately calmed down and proceeded to get on her toy car and push the button that played a horrible-sounding (to me) "Care Bear" tune that clearly didn't bother her! Cow out, bear in. The logic was a difficult code to crack.

Despite this diversity in clinical presentations, what many autism symptoms have in common is that they are consistent with a dysfunctional glutamatergic network, and in fact glutamatergic dysfunction is widely recognized as a central mechanism in autism.[26] This understanding is consistent with thinking about autism in terms of E/I imbalance. Recall that the E refers to *excitatory* signaling (which is glutamate-based) and the I refers to *inhibitory* signaling (which is GABA-based). In a healthy mind and body, the excitatory system is balanced by the inhibitory system, and the stimulating function of glutamate is balanced by the calming effects of GABA.[27]

The basic observation that links autism to glutamate dysregulation is an abnormally high number of glutamate receptors in the cerebellum of autism patients.[28] The cerebellum is the area of the brain responsible for sensory and motor activity. This is a critical finding because glutamate receptors are essential players in the neural networking of the brain, and critical to learning and memory.[29] Alterations of this neural wiring is observed in the brains of autism patients and explains the atypical neural development associated with autism symptoms.[30]

Another piece of the autism puzzle that has led scientists to the autism–glutamate connection is the discovery of certain molecules in the blood and urine samples of autism patients. These metabolites are often produced by cells responding to toxic levels of glutamate, and bear the signatures of inflammation, oxidative stress, and cell damage.[31] This metabolic panel is what I would expect with glutamate dysregulation playing a role in autism.[32] Unfortunately, these metabolites can indicate other diseases as well as autism and, alone, cannot be used for a diagnosis.

What about the gut–brain connection? More than 70 percent of those diagnosed with autism have intestinal symptoms. This is not part of the autism diagnosis—yet. Since I started writing this section, more scientific attention has been focused on the gut and the microbiome's association with autism spectrum disorder. Within the digestive tract are a wide array of glutamate receptors and many gut–brain neural connections, and for some with autism, glutamate-mediated aberrant signaling may have its origin in the gut. Whether the cause or a consequence, it is a fact that digestive issues, microbial changes, and metabolic imbalance are common features of the autism profile.[33]

My experience with Taylor tells me that what one eats makes a difference in autism, but I am not the only person who has seen this.

Harvard researcher and autism expert Martha Herbert was an early advocate of a whole food, MSG-free diet to support brain health. In her book, *The Autism Revolution: Whole Body Strategies for Making Life All It Can Be*,[34] Herbert chronicles changes she observed when her patients adopted a nutrient-dense, plant-based diet and avoided ingesting excitotoxins such as monosodium glutamate (MSG) in their food. In some patients, the health benefits were so profound that autism symptoms disappeared altogether.

Cancer

No other cell type is characterized by more metabolic dysfunction than cancer cells. Cancer is deadly and widespread. The American Cancer Society projected that in 2022, 1,762,450 new cancer cases and 606,880 cancer deaths would occur in the United States that year alone.[35] Worldwide, the think tank GlobeScan reported 18.1 million new cases of cancer and 9.6 million deaths from cancer in 2018.[36]

Cancer cells can be found in tissues throughout the body and in blood. Cancer cells arise from normal cells, but they have different characteristics from normal cells. In particular, cancers exhibit uncontrolled cell division and growth. The more rapid the abnormal cell growth is, the more aggressive and damaging the cancer. In the decades spent characterizing cancers, understanding how cancer cells grow and invade tissues has been the focus of much research.

Rapid cell growth requires readily accessible, generous sources of energy. Glucose is by far the molecule most often utilized for energy in our cells, and cancer cells feed their high energy needs by ramping up their use of glucose. The amplification of glucose utilization in tumors is the science behind how PET scans detect cancer. But cancer cells' demand for energy can be satisfied by glutamate, too. Hungry cancer cells will consume glutamate if it is available, and if it is not, they will make glutamate from other molecules such as glutamine, a common nutritional supplement.

It turns out that glutamate is a handy molecule for cancer cells to have around for other reasons. A cancer cell with excess glutamate will secrete glutamate, and this has been shown to stimulate tumor growth, proliferation, and survival of other cancer cells. Glutamate secreted by cancer cells can also kill nearby healthy cells. Nowhere is this scenario more apparent and dangerous than in the brain. In addition to their demand for energy, cancer cells also need room to grow, and in the brain, space is limited by the rigid skull bone. To solve the problem, some cancer cells simply poison their healthy neighbors by releasing glutamate. The excitotoxic effect of elevated glutamate on normal cells causes an influx of calcium into brain cells, leading to cell death. The death of normal cells then provides room for cancer cells to grow and spread.[37] Various types of cancer cells have been shown to kill normal cells by releasing glutamate and increasing glutamate signaling in the area surrounding them.[38] With the death of normal cells, cancer cells invade.

It gets worse. Normal cells sometimes respond to the glutamate bath created by cancerous tumor cells by increasing the number of glutamate receptors on their cell surfaces, transforming their properties in such a way as to enable them to participate in—*and benefit from*—the glutamatergic signaling initiated by the cancer. Can't beat them? Join them. The transformation of healthy cells into cancer cells, as they respond to the elevated levels of glutamate in their environment, is likely the mechanism promoting many cancers.[39]

Recall that inflammation and cancer are connected. As described in chapter 6, "The Slow-Growing Fire: Inflammation and Diet," one of the ways a cell communicates stress is through the release of glutamate. If a cell is highly stressed, it can release so much glutamate that it ignites something researchers call a *cytokine storm*. Cytokines are substances released by the body's immune cells to ensure that a protective inflammatory/immune response is mounted. However, a cytokine storm is more than that—think of a cytokine storm as a glutamate stress signal so overblown that it is dangerous. This is doubly concerning because such a signal is the same signal that cancer cells use to recruit nearby healthy cells into the ranks of cancer cells. In other words, the very signals cells use to communicate a stress or inflammatory response[40] have been linked to the transformation of cells to a cancer-like metabolism, and to tumor growth.[41] Chronic inflammation, then, provides a pathway for the initiation and propagation of cancer.

The medical research community widely recognizes that glutamate and glutamatergic signaling are players in the initiation, proliferation, and survival of cancers. Consistent with this thread of research, doctors are increasingly prescribing glutamate antagonists (blockers) to treat many types of cancers.

Depression

Depression is a persistent feeling of sadness and loss of interests that affects how a person feels, thinks, and behaves, which can lead to a variety of emotional and physical problems. Glutamate imbalance plays a role in depression, as it does in many mood disorders.[42] Underlying these disorders is inflammation and aberrant glutamate signaling.

How does that work? In effect, the abnormal signal from misfiring nerve cells causes inflammation (and nerve cells can be misfiring for any reason—disease, diet, or external events, to name a few). This adds noise to the nervous system, such that the normal glutamate signaling coming from routine activities of daily life is now distorted. This reverberates throughout the nervous system, and you just don't feel well.

Fortunately, much research has focused on the links between inflammation, depression, and maladaptive glutamate signaling.[43] One result of this research has been to identify a subcategory of depression specifically referred to as glutamate-based depression (GBD), which comes about when disease or environmental stress disrupts normal glutamatergic signaling.

As one group of researchers states,

> Ample evidence now indicates that glutamate homeostasis and neurotransmission are disrupted in major depressive disorder. . . . We define glutamate-based depression (GBD) as a chronic depressive illness associated with environmental stress and diseases associated with altered glutamate neurotransmission. GBD provides an underlying biological mechanism for the high incidence of depression in these diseases.[44]

In plain language, these researchers are saying that glutamate-based depression and diseases associated with chronic inflammation are inextricably linked. Diseases associated with high rates of glutamate-based depression include coronary heart disease, Alzheimer's disease, diabetes, Parkinson's disease, Huntington's disease, fibromyalgia, rheumatoid arthritis, and chronic pain. Unfortunately, even after the triggering inflammatory insult has been resolved (for example, you overcame a COVID-19 infection), the glutamatergic neural rewiring that occurred when you were inflamed still exerts an effect (you have lingering pain or brain fog, as in long COVID, which I posit is a residual effect of the reworking of your glutamatergic network). In other words, you may be managing the disease, but the new, altered glutamate receptor map is still part of your makeup, and its energy demands can exhaust you. It can leave you feeling listless—a classic symptom of depression.

Because of this insight, glutamate antagonists (blockers) are increasingly prescribed for treating depression. The focus of treatment? Reducing glutamate neurotransmission. That's why these medications are referred to as glutamate blocker drugs. It's also the reason why so many sufferers with depression are able to reduce symptoms with dietary changes, including adoption of the REID food lifestyle.

Diabetes, Obesity, and Metabolic Syndrome

To most people, the term "metabolism" is a broad term describing how their body obtains energy from the foods they eat. People say, "I have a high metabolism," or "Exercise increases my metabolism and gives me more energy." That is the big picture. What is not so often thought about is the *metabolism of one's individual cells*, but this is where disease and the body's energy needs intersect.

As described in the section on cancer, a hallmark of diseased cells is a metabolism that is out of whack. This can be detected through a wide variety of medical tests available today. Major health issues causing widespread suffering in modern societies—metabolic syndrome, diabetes, obesity—can all be classified as energy imbalance disorders. At the root of each disorder are cells in which the normal metabolic functions are in disarray. Since glutamate is involved in a large number of metabolic reactions *inside* the cell (in addition to signaling *between* cells), it's not surprising that glutamate dysregulation and energy imbalance go hand in hand.

Diabetes

Diabetes (*diabetes mellitus*) is a group of metabolic diseases (the most common being Type 2 diabetes) in which the body's ability to produce or respond to the hormone insulin is impaired. This results in too much glucose (sugar) in the blood and urine, and too little in our cells, which then can become starved for energy. Those that suffer the disease often experience increased thirst, urination, and appetite. In 2022, the CDC estimated that more than 130 million U.S. adults are living with diabetes or pre-diabetes.[45] Diabetes is a classic example of energy imbalance, and it has to do with the body's inability to regulate glucose.

What does it mean to say that the body cannot regulate glucose? The first thing to know is that, even though glucose is the main source of energy for human cells, it can't enter our cells without help. Glucose isn't simply absorbed by hungry cells; instead, it needs to be actively transported into the cell through special "gates" in the cell membrane. These gates open when insulin binds to insulin receptors in the cell membrane—think key (insulin) in the keyhole (insulin receptor) popping open the door (enter glucose). In this way, insulin acts as the gatekeeper, allowing glucose to enter the cell. Timing is critical, though. Usually, insulin is released by the pancreas after we eat. This means our cells open up their gates to receive their meal of glucose at the exact moment when glucose is present in the blood. Our energy needs are thus met, synchronized with our ingestion of food. At least, that is how it is supposed to work.

What is often not considered in the diabetes story is the major role glutamate plays in this disease. It turns out that glutamate—not blood glucose—is what controls the release of insulin from the pancreas. Looking at excess glutamate as the cause of insulin dysregulation requires a different approach to diabetes that is not yet fully appreciated by the medical industry.

Why is glutamate the key player here? In the pancreas, there exists a type of cell called beta cells (aka β-cells), and these are the cells that secrete insulin. Glutamate controls the flow of insulin from beta cells. The more glutamate in the pancreas, the more insulin released into the blood—sometimes without regard to the body's blood glucose level. This can lead to chronically elevated insulin, which is the recipe for an energy imbalance.

Cells respond to chronically elevated insulin by reducing the number of gates that allow glucose to pass into the cell. The cell can also shut down gates by making the gates less sensitive to insulin. That means more insulin is required for the gates to open. In practice, cells do both things when exposed to too much insulin. This is the fundamental cause of *insulin resistance*, which is one of the defining characteristics of Type 2 diabetes. The consequence of insulin resistance is that cells shut down the glucose gates, even while, paradoxically, they may be hungry for glucose. Again, a recipe for an energy imbalance.

Elevated insulin levels set other things in motion, too. Various feedback signals send the message to the pancreas to stop producing insulin. This message gets garbled in the presence of excess glutamate signaling and chronic activation of the glutamate receptors on beta cells. The result is that beta cells continue to produce insulin—the insulin faucet is wide open. Ultimately, chronic activation of beta cells can prove toxic. Beta cells get sick or die off, and the pancreas stops making insulin—not because it got the message to stop making insulin, but because it is no longer able to do so.

How does insulin resistance impact the brain? The brain has a major requirement for energy—approximately 20 percent of your total available energy is used by the brain. Glucose is the major supplier of this energy, and brain cells can become insulin resistant, too. Insulin-resistant brain cells don't fare well. When starved of energy, neurons can lose function, causing major deficits in memory and cognition. This can lead to diseases such as dementia and Alzheimer's.

The surprising association between insulin resistance and an entire suite of diseases has brought new insights into the mechanisms of disease, including Alzheimer's. In fact, Alzheimer's disease is sometimes referred to as Type 3 diabetes. The impact of insulin dysregulation also might be the underlying reason many people with unmanaged Type 2 diabetes experience cognitive issues (think brain fog). Is it possible to have Alzheimer's without being diagnosed with Type 2 diabetes? Yes. Because of the brain's high energy requirement, insulin resistance in the brain may occur (along with the deficits associated with Alzheimer's) before a metabolic issue is detected elsewhere in the body.

One thing to keep in mind is that nearly all the metabolic adjustments that our bodies make are in the service of maintaining homeostasis—the body's status quo. When the insulin faucet is dysregulated or broken, our entire body has to adapt to the reality of too much glucose circulating in the blood, and no reliable way to get this important energy molecule into hungry cells.

As for the starving cells that have become unresponsive to insulin, they satisfy their energy requirements by using alternative sources of energy, such as fat. This is resourceful, but has unfortunate downstream consequences. The increased demand for fat causes adipose tissue to release fat in the form of triglycerides. Triglycerides get dumped into the blood, which then transports the triglycerides to energy-starved cells. Triglycerides, then, become the cell's go-to molecule for energy. Now we have an imbalance in fat metabolism, which can lead to dyslipidemia, or fat metabolism dysregulation. In a chain reaction of dysfunction, what was a case of glucose dysregulation has ballooned into a case of fat dysregulation.

Given the widespread occurrence of diabetes across modern society, and the understanding that this disease is highly correlated with blood glutamate levels,[46] it is imperative to support scientific research that examines the role our newfound addiction to glutamate plays in the origin of these enormous health problems. Until that happens, one way to empower yourself is to eat whole foods, avoid processed food, and remove enriched sources of glutamate from your diet.

Obesity

In modern societies, there is an epidemic of health issues stemming from food abundance. The CDC statistics on obesity are staggering, if not immediately obvious to anyone walking out their door. As of 2017–2018, 42.4 percent of the U.S. adult population was obese, and nearly three-fourths of American adults were overweight or obese.[47]

At issue is not *all* food, however; it's the quantity of the *wrong kind of food* available on our overstocked shelves that is making us sick.

Obesity is defined as having a body mass index score (BMI) of 30.0 or greater. This excess weight is the physical expression of an energy imbalance: the body has to deal with the presence of too much energy, and it stores it as fat. Simply put, consuming more calories than you use results in weight gain. However, other factors are at play, such as the hormone *leptin*.

Have you ever felt that you can't lose weight, even though you have cut your intake of calories? Leptin (and in particular, leptin dysregulation) may be the culprit sabotaging your efforts. We have to go back to our prehistoric ancestors to understand why, evolutionarily, leptin exists at all. There was a time—actually, that "time" is anytime in the human record that isn't now—when getting enough calories was difficult. Our survival as a species was dependent on weathering the lean times, and leptin helps us do that by adjusting our metabolic rate. When there are not enough calories to go around, leptin turns down our metabolic engine so that fewer calories are needed.

The problem for modern societies arises when leptin becomes dysregulated. In this case, there's a disconnect in the leptin signaling pathway, and it is no longer correlated with what you eat. If you cut calories, leptin may very well in turn reduce your metabolic rate *and* direct glucose to be stored as fat. What effect would this have on an individual? It would be like going on a diet to lose weight, but you don't lose weight. Instead, you feel a lack of energy as your body socks away calories for the future. And just like glutamate is at the heart of insulin dysregulation, glutamate is at the heart of leptin dysregulation.

Here's the background: leptin is a hormone derived from adipose (fat) tissue. This hormone can cross the blood-brain barrier, where it acts on leptin receptors in the hypothalamus and hippocampus regions of the brain. These structures are the major control centers responsible for hunger, thirst, sleep, emotions, memory, and learning. Leptin is often referred to as a satiety hormone because it balances energy by controlling our desire to eat and determining the amount of energy to store as fat. When leptin binds to leptin receptors in the brain, we feel full.

Now glutamate steps in. In the same way that glutamate controls insulin release in the pancreas, glutamate regulates leptin release from fat cells. This is the truly insidious way glutamate makes you fat. When excess glutamate is circulating, leptin metabolism can become dysregulated, making brain cells leptin resistant. This means that after a meal, *even if significant levels of leptin are present in the blood*, your brain doesn't get the message that you have had your fill because neurons are not registering the "full" signal. So you keep eating, wanting more and more food in order to feel full.

For decades, research scientists have understood that excess glutamate causes obesity via its role in leptin regulation. If you still have doubts, think about this: the pharmaceutical industry is in constant need of a supply of obese rats and mice to test various drugs for treating obesity. How are these obese animals created? In addition to feeding lab animals MSG-laced food, as described earlier in this book, another tried and true way is through injection of glutamate.[48] The important point here is that animals injected with MSG are not consuming more calories. They become obese because glutamate is disrupting their metabolic rate. The connection between MSG load and obesity has also been documented in numerous human population studies.[49] In one study, long-term MSG consumption has been found to disrupt normal appetite regulation, resulting in obesity and shorter stature in individuals. The researchers were alarmed by this finding and offered this warning:

> The present study for the first time demonstrates that a widely used nutritional [substance]—the flavouring agent MSG—at concentrations that only slightly surpass those found in everyday human food, exhibits significant potential for damaging the hypothalamic regulation of appetite, and thereby determines the propensity of world-wide obesity. We suggest to reconsider the recommended daily allowances of amino acids and nutritional protein, and to abstain from the popular protein-rich diets, and particularly from adding the flavouring agents MSG.[50]

What the study's authors are saying is that the widespread use of MSG as a food additive has the potential for causing obesity on a global scale. This concern prompts them to ask food governing bodies to reconsider the current daily recommended allowances of amino acids and nutritional protein (foods that are sources of MSG), and to advocate abstinence from MSG. This study was done in 2006. No action was taken. This is greatly concerning because today, MSG and processed foods are an even larger part of modern diets, and the current amount of MSG in everyday human food certainly exceeds what these authors estimated then.

Metabolic Syndrome

Metabolic syndrome is characterized by the co-occurrence of certain cardiovascular risk factors, including obesity, insulin resistance, and high blood pressure. The connection between cardiovascular disease and energy imbalance issues is straightforward.

Recall that when excess blood glucose is converted to fat and stored in adipose tissue, there is an uptick in blood triglycerides. Triglycerides remain elevated when cells can't effectively use glucose for energy and instead demand new energy sources from fat. The consequence of this shift in cell metabolism, from glucose-burning to fat-burning, is an excess of triglycerides in the bloodstream. Fatty blood, fatty liver, and a fatty vascular system ensue—conditions that open the door to cardiovascular disease.

The notion that glutamate in the food supply is directly linked to diabetes, obesity, metabolic syndrome,[51] and cardiovascular disease is not a new idea.[52] Despite the preponderance of evidence, the glutamate industry aggressively attacks research that establishes these links,[53] successfully undermining public awareness of the issue. Yet scientists are still asking questions. If you only scan the titles of the scientific reports cited in this chapter in the "Notes" section at the end of this book, you will get a sense of where this line of research is heading, who is connecting the dots, and what we know so far.

Multiple Sclerosis

Multiple sclerosis (MS) is an autoimmune disease that attacks the proteins that make up the myelin sheath, a protective layer surrounding the main stem or axon of a neuron. Symptoms include muscle weakness, spasms, fatigue, and numbness in various parts of the body. Unfortunately, MS symptoms can manifest as any neurological disorder and is often misdiagnosed. In the United States, over 1 million people live with MS, and there are 2.3 million sufferers worldwide.[54]

The general consensus among researchers is that multiple sclerosis begins with the formation of acute inflammatory lesions, which damage the neuron's protective myelin coat. The slow erosion of the myelin sheath, called demyelination, results in the breakdown of neuronal signaling and is the cause of MS's debilitating symptoms. MS is considered an inflammatory disease because the damage to the nerve cell is due to chronically elevated levels of glutamate. In fact, *glutamate-induced cell damage* is likely the underlying mechanism explaining the symptoms associated with the disease.

As one set of researchers stated,

> Research advances support the idea that excessive activation of the glutamatergic pathway plays an important part in the pathophysiology of multiple sclerosis. Beyond the well-established direct toxic effects on neurons, additional sites of glutamate-induced cell damage have been described, including effects in oligodendrocytes, astrocytes, endothelial cells, and immune cells. Such toxic effects could provide a link between various pathological aspects of multiple sclerosis, such as axonal damage, oligodendrocyte cell death, demyelination, autoimmunity, and blood-brain barrier dysfunction.[55]

While elevated glutamate and increased number of glutamate receptors in the brain are hallmarks of the disease,[56] numerous studies over two decades also make clear the relationship between elevated glutamate and the progression and severity of MS symptoms.[57] One team of researchers used magnetic resonance imaging (MRI) to follow 265 MS patients and the progression of their disease over an average of 1.8 years. They found what is now well-established: a significant positive correlation between elevated glutamate levels and increased neurodegeneration.[58]

While a low-inflammatory diet has long been touted to help manage MS symptoms,[59] we need to be better educated about what exactly *is* a low-inflammatory diet. This may mean different foods for different people. Based on what we know now, a good place to start would be to avoid all sources of enriched glutamate from foods and beverages. In other words, don't eat factory processed foods.

Parkinson's Disease (Parkinsonism)

Parkinson's disease is a progressive, neurodegenerative disorder thought to affect more than 4 million people worldwide.[60] The onset of symptoms usually happens late in life. Some of the core motor symptoms of Parkinson's are loss of voluntary movement, rigidity, resting tremor, and postural and balance difficulties. This is experienced as difficulty buttoning a shirt, moving fluidly across a dance floor, or playing the piano. Patients can also suffer from a broad spectrum of non-motor symptoms. Men are 1.5 times more likely to be afflicted with Parkinson's disease than women.

Like so many diseases involving glutamate, Parkinson's is characterized by aberrant glutamate signaling. Glutamate signaling is essential in the control of movement, starting in the brain. This signaling allows the thought "I want to pick up a coffee cup" to become action by translating your intention to the muscles in your arm and hand. Your glutamate receptor map creates the body awareness that allows your hand to guide the coffee cup to your mouth with precision. With Parkinson's, the glutamate signal isn't translated effectively, due to damage to a group of neurons deep at the base of the brain called the basal ganglia. The basal ganglia is part of our sensory system and, when these neurons misfire, there is a mismatch between what you intend to do and what your body actually does.

What does this look like? On a cellular level, the disease is characterized by over-stimulation of glutamate receptors and excess glutamate signaling of neurons.[61] On a personal level, instead of smoothly picking up your coffee cup, you experience involuntary movement and tremors in the hand holding the coffee cup. You have to really think about getting the coffee cup to your lips without spilling it.

The neurotransmitter dopamine has long been the focus of Parkinson's disease research because one of the biomarkers of the disorder is the degeneration of dopamine receptors on neurons. However, what is not often recognized in considering this aspect of the disease is how dopamine metabolism is regulated by glutamate. (Recall that the relationship between glutamate and dopamine was also mentioned with respect to addiction and ADHD.) In Parkinson's, glutamate excitotoxicity damages dopamine receptors, causing a drop in dopamine.[62] In an ever-worsening feedback loop, when dopamine levels drop, neurons are even more vulnerable to glutamate excitotoxicity, leading to progression of the disease.[63]

Today, we have a greater understanding of how diet and our own microbiome are involved in neurotransmitter balance, and how food choices may help in delaying the onset and progression of neurological diseases like Parkinson's. More needs to be done. This was the conclusion of a 2018 study investigating the role of dietary neurotransmitters in neurological diseases. These researchers also recommended that dietary approaches be considered in treating a wide variety of neurological disorders.[64]

Schizophrenia

Schizophrenia is a brain disorder that alters the way a person thinks, acts, and perceives the world. At worst, the disconnect between what a person experiences and what is real results in a significant loss of contact with reality. Before the onset of severe symptoms, many will experience cognitive deficits like poor memory, "brain fog," and poor attention span. Nearly 1 percent of the U.S. population is diagnosed with schizophrenia.

The best explanation for the wide variety of symptoms displayed in schizophrenia, as in most diseases, is that the pathology is rooted in inflammation. Those afflicted with schizophrenia are much more likely to have an early health history of frequent immune activation and chronic inflammation.[65] Examples of chronic inflammation in children are eczema or other persistent rashes, moderate to severe asthma, and many environmental allergies. Examples of immune activation events include moderate to severe infections (think strep, mononucleosis, ear infections), trauma, and auto-immune disorders, including immune reactions to foods, as in celiac disease.

The food connection is particularly relevant to our discussion here. For some people, schizophrenia is associated with serum antibodies against dietary antigens, such as gliadin (a component of gluten), and casein,[66] the proteins found in wheat and dairy, respectively. As a personal aside, after my TEDx talk on the hazards of glutamate in foods, a woman in her 60s emailed me, sharing her story. As a young adult, Beth was diagnosed with schizophrenia and believed it was a diagnosis she would carry for the rest of her life. At the age of 60, she started experimenting with her diet for other health reasons and eliminated many foods, including wheat and dairy. She said that after changing her diet, she no longer experienced schizophrenic episodes—something she had lived with for nearly 40 years! Her story resonated with me, given my journey with Taylor and my work with so many clients. Finding the root cause of inflammation, particularly with food choices that we absolutely can control, can change your life.

What is happening on the cellular level, such that glutamate and schizophrenia should be linked? It is postulated that an early immune activation event,[67] which results in a person being more vulnerable to glutamate excitotoxicity, could set the stage for later development of the disorder. Whatever its origins, brain imaging of patients, postmortem analysis of brain tissue, and animal studies point to damage to neurons by glutamate dysregulation as the underlying cause of the symptoms in schizophrenia.[68]

Interestingly, what led researchers to investigate the role of glutamate in schizophrenia was the observation that the glutamate blocker drugs ketamine and PCP (phencyclidine) produced symptoms that mirrored schizophrenia. Ketamine—a powerful anesthetic with the street name "Special K"—is known for its hallucinogenic dissociative properties, making it useful in surgeries and a party drug favorite. The behaviors of PCP drug addicts so matched those of schizophrenic patients that some PCP drug addicts were mistakenly diagnosed with schizophrenia. Such is the evidence of the complex role of glutamate dysregulation in this psychiatric condition.[69]

Seizures/Epilepsy

Epilepsy is characterized either by mild, episodic loss of attention or sleepiness, or—the version most of us know from movies—instances marked by severe convulsions and loss of consciousness.

The lineup of players implicated in epilepsy are names we have heard before. Neurochemical markers of epilepsy in blood plasma include abnormal concentrations of the amino acids glutamate, aspartate, and glycine.[70] Glutamate receptors have been implicated in inducing epileptic convulsions through overstimulation of glutamate-activated ion portals.[71] Mechanically, it works this way: when glutamate binds to the glutamate receptors on a nerve cell, the sodium and calcium ion gates open. This increases nerve activity. The abnormal functioning of these ion gates plays an integral role in causing seizures. In fact, this abnormal functioning can be visualized on an EEG of the brain of epilepsy sufferers.

When it comes to food . . . well, you don't hear much about diet and avoiding glutamate to help with seizure management. This is baffling, since the initial goal of a ketogenic diet (high-fat, low carbohydrate), developed in the 1920s, was to improve the balance in glutamate signaling in the brains of epilepsy patients, and thereby alleviate seizures.[72]

A change in diet was the approach I took in one case involving a young boy who was having frequent seizures. Ethan had been adopted as a baby and his biological mother was a meth addict. Gail, his adopted mother, reached out to me in a panic after Ethan was admitted to Stanford Hospital following a particularly terrifying seizure. At the time he was nine years old. My food recommendations required an overhaul of family meals so that they consisted of a balance of whole foods, which are critical for managing blood glucose and glutamate levels. I also stressed the importance of squash seeds and dark green leafy vegetables such as kale and parsley as natural sources of magnesium, which is often supplemented in epileptic patients. It was a lifesaving change for the boy and his family. The seizures, which had been weekly, were now separated by months at a time. Today Ethan is 13. Gail still occasionally consults with me regarding her other adopted children and has let me know that Ethan is doing better. He loves hiking.

Other Neurodegenerative Disorders

There's a host of other neuroinflammatory diseases that result in aberrant glutamate signaling, and many more that are rare genetic conditions leading to glutamate dysregulation.[73] The mechanisms of disease vary, and can involve autoimmune factors (antibodies binding to glutamate receptors or proteins involved in glutamate metabolism), genetic mutations in glutamate receptors, and chronic inflammation. The point here is that these conditions are exacerbated by a lifestyle that increases glutamate signaling and metabolism. And the question we should all be asking ourselves is: why are these disorders increasing in modern societies at alarming rates?

Here I've provided a partial list of additional glutamate dysregulation-based diseases. Some conditions on this list will be unfamiliar to most; others are well-known to just about everyone. I've included short descriptions of a few conditions, with references, that didn't quite make it into the main body of this chapter but are of keen interest to many readers.

- AIDS dementia complex
- Amyotrophic lateral sclerosis (Lou Gehrig's disease)
- Arthritis
- Combined systems disease (vitamin B12 deficiency)
- Fibromyalgia (a chronic disorder characterized by widespread musculoskeletal pain, fatigue, and tenderness in localized areas). Two dietary studies reported marked improvements in symptoms after removing glutamate-rich foods.[74]
- Glaucoma
- Huntington's disease (a genetic disorder caused by mutations in the huntingtin [*HTT*] gene, which results in neurodegeneration. The *HTT* gene is involved in the packaging and transport of glutamate inside vesicles within the cell; mutations in the gene alter glutamate trafficking). Glutamate excitotoxicity is one the main mechanisms of progression of neurodegeneration.
- Immune deficiency
- Inflamed skin (i.e., eczema)
- Ischemia (the technical term describing any condition where there is an insufficient blood supply to your tissues and organs; stroke—lack of blood flow to the brain—is perhaps the most familiar example of ischemia)

- Lead encephalopathy
- Migraines (experienced as a recurrent throbbing headache, often accompanied by sensory sensitivities to sound or light, nausea, and vomiting). Many people report food as a trigger of migraines, with MSG being one of the most common triggers reported. Diet has been shown to help manage symptoms.[75] Inflammation (and its compeer, glutamate dysregulation) is believed to be an underlying condition that makes a person more susceptible to migraines.[76]
- Mitochondrial abnormalities (and other inherited or acquired biochemical disorders)
- Neuropathic pain syndromes (e.g., causalgia or painful peripheral neuropathies)
- Essential tremor
- Restless leg syndrome
- Rett's syndrome
- Wernicke's encephalopathy

The Takeaway

The diseases and disorders described in this chapter have a common underlying mechanism—glutamate dysregulation. Glutamate in the diet has the potential to exacerbate any of these conditions by adding fuel to the fire. The 1959 FDA designation that glutamate is "Generally Recognized As Safe" is grossly out of date in today's world of processed food and our modern understanding of human health, but so far Big Food has had little incentive to stop making glutamate-enriched products that are enormously profitable and consumers find addicting.

So, what do we do about this? Read on—next is the antidote.

Roadmap to Health

THE REID FOOD LIFESTYLE

BOOKS ADVOCATING VARIOUS FOOD LIFESTYLES AS THE WAY TO OP-
timal health crowd bookstore shelves. Vegan, vegetarian, paleo, keto,
low-fat, low-carb, good carb . . . recipes for wellness are everywhere.
You might think all these approaches would advocate eliminating or
reducing commercially processed foods in the diet. Amazingly, many
popular diet books and nutrition gurus don't make a big deal about this.
REID does make a big deal about eliminating commercially processed
foods, but still . . . absent these foods, what is special about REID that
makes it different from everything else you've read?

The REID (Reduced Excitatory Inflammatory Diet) food lifestyle considers food's impact on health at the *molecular* level. REID
is based in biochemistry. Its food recommendations are predicated on
the awareness that one substance, glutamate—which is present in large
amounts in processed food—is indisputably linked to chronic inflammatory diseases. REID names the sources of glutamate in food, and in
doing so gives readers specific guidance for what to eat, and what not
to eat. Think of REID as a journey to *redefine* food. That's a break from
past diets that only counted calories or simply advised us to eat one
kind of food over another.

I'll start by describing the six principles that form the foundation of
REID. Then, to help you implement this new food lifestyle, I give you 10
goals and steps. This chapter, along with appendix B, "The Perfect Plate:

Recipes, Ingredients, and Meal Plans," will help you visualize yourself in places where you must make critical decisions: at the grocery store, in your kitchen, and at your favorite social events. Navigate the food aisles, family mealtimes, and the buffet table with confidence—you've got this!

REID Principles

Principle 1: Reduce Excitotoxicity

Excitotoxicity refers to the process whereby a chemical excites or activates a cell to death. Glutamate is by far the most abundant excitotoxin in the food supply, but there are others, such as aspartate, aspartame (an artificial sweetener), cysteine, and glutamine. REID reduces your exposure to glutamate and other excitotoxins and can help return your nervous system to a healthy state.

As figure 8.1 illustrates, keeping glutamate levels low is key to keeping inflammation in check.

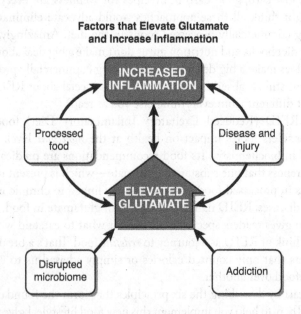

Figure 8.1 There are many ways glutamate levels in the body can be elevated. All lead to inflammation.

Preexisting health conditions, from minor pollen allergies to serious disorders like autism and Parkinson's disease, may render a person particularly sensitive to the excitotoxic effects of even low levels of glutamate. A sensitive individual may have a baseline inflammation that is already so high that the simple act of eating common foods off the grocery shelf will seriously worsen excitatory symptoms. That's why some people are more sensitive to glutamate in the diet than others.

Principle 2: Reduce Inflammation

Each person's inflammation load is unique, even among family members. Unfortunately, there are many foods that can induce inflammation, and any one individual's vulnerability can be impacted by personal food sensitivities/allergies, metabolic and immune challenges, and genetic factors. That said, some foods, such as those with chemical additives, added sugar, or low in fiber, are inflammatory to just about everybody. REID will help lower your own inflammation bucket (or that of affected loved ones) by showing you how to avoid those foods. You are then encouraged to see for yourself which foods might contribute to your individual inflammation bucket. The food journey is personal.

Principle 3: Increase Fiber from Vegetables

Leafy and high-fiber vegetables form the foundations of the REID food pyramid (figure 8.2). REID raises fiber to the level of a macronutrient in its own right, not a subcategory under carbohydrate, as traditionally defined. Think of fiber as a SUPER-macronutrient—it is that important to health. There is no such thing as "indigestible starch" when we consider the energy extracted from these foods by the microbes in our intestines.

In its food recommendations, REID considers the ratio of nutrients in the diet and how this affects not just humans but also the microbial ecosystem in our digestive tract. Both microbes and human cells need to be fed a diverse and balanced plate of whole foods. When the proportion of high-fiber vegetables, such as asparagus, broccoli, celery, fennel, and kale, far exceeds the proportion of proteins and fats taken

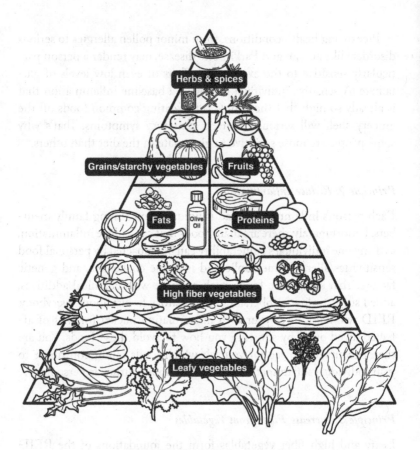

Figure 8.2 The REID food pyramid.

in, the environment of the large intestine supports healthy microbial communities, which in turn promote our health.

How does that work? If microbes in the large intestine are not given fiber, they will instead ferment protein and fats, which is associated with inflammation. In our protein-obsessed food culture, where the food label "added protein" increases sales, REID seeks to tip the scales away from added protein in favor of vegetable fiber.

Another point: we want to choose our foods so that we achieve maximum fermentation in the large intestine, not the small intestine.

REID advocates a wide variety of herbs and bitter foods that naturally discourage fermentation in the small intestine, where microbial over-growth can occur. See appendix B for strategies to help you get there.

Principle 4: Diversify!

Variety, variety, variety is the name of the game here. If you never ate celery root or had dandelion tea, well then, a new day provides an op-portunity to try something novel. A variety of beautiful, new whole foods in your diet will best meet your energy needs, allowing your ner-vous system to rewire and reduce your risk for disease. Wellness is built from the inside out. Try different foods, and your body will get and use what it requires.

Principle 5: Know Where Your Food Comes from and How It's Made

We won't learn everything about a food product by reading labels, but it's a good place to start. REID avoids foods listing vague ingredients such as "natural flavors," which can consist of any of thousands of pos-sible chemicals. The only flavors in your meal should come from the foods themselves, and those herbs.

Principle 6: Embrace the Food Journey as a Lifestyle

Resisting, denying, or doubting that foods can be healing, or—what's worse—surrendering to an inflammatory health condition as just "it is what it is"—can stop you in your tracks. Embrace the food journey as something exciting and new. We are individuals, and as in any adventure, there are things to be learned. Find what works for you and your family.

With these principles in mind, let's set some goals.

Putting REID into Practice: 10 Goals

Here are 10 goals to help guide you on your way. The key to success is your mindset—your resolve to do what is necessary for the health of your family.

Goal 1: A *Call to Action* to redefine food
Goal 2: Eliminate wheat gluten and processed grains
Goal 3: Eliminate dairy
Goal 4: Increase consumption of high-fiber vegetables and herbs throughout the day
Goal 5: Clean out your environment (start with your kitchen)
Goal 6: Restock your kitchen
Goal 7: Eliminate refined sugars and reserve fruit as a treat
Goal 8: Identify your go-to foods
Goal 9: Have a quality control plan for consuming foods outside the home
Goal 10: Embrace the journey toward the perfect plate

Goal 1: A **Call to Action** *to Redefine Food*

For many, and certainly for my family, this lifestyle journey meant redefining food. This goal is more of a mental preparation and requires understanding that real food comes from the ground, or in the case of animals, is taken from the sea or raised in a humane manner in a natural environment with the animal's natural diet. When initially defining your family's foods, the first question usually is "what do we eat?" I know that you may be asking yourself, "how am I going to get my picky eater to eat fennel and chard?" It can be done, and I will show you how. Remember: there are many battles we face in our lifetime, and this one is worth fighting. We, and especially our children, are in a war zone, where processed foods are everywhere, enticing us to consume. The sooner you start fighting back, the sooner healthy eating becomes a habit and part of your core family values.

Step 1: Be passionate about improving your and your family's health through food. Be patient. Remind yourself that although change can be challenging, the reward of wellness is worth the effort (even if the kids bewail their favorite cookies being banned from the house).

Step 2: Encourage the troops. Talk about the importance of eating healthy food.

- Explain how we use food to nourish our bodies. Some foods make us feel well and strong, while other foods can make us feel ill, too tired, too high energy, or even make us feel hungrier.
- Encourage family members to talk about how certain foods make them feel. Ask yourself: when I eat _____, I feel _____. Remember: your gut talks to your brain, and how you feel may be telling you whether a food is excitatory. This is most effective at the beginning, when processed foods may not have been completely eliminated from the diet.

Step 3: Arm yourself. REID is all about incorporating a variety of whole foods, and investing in some basic kitchen tools helps the mission. The following are not required, but together they make the REID journey easier.

- Stainless steel pots and pans and a good set of knives are basic tools.
- A high-powered blender like Vitamix® or Nutrabullet® makes it easier to incorporate whole foods into smoothies, sauces, soups, dressings, batters, dips, and salsas. I have used the Vitamix every day since I first invested in this accessory. I even take it camping, and sometimes when I travel. It is indispensable.
- A simple grinder like a coffee grinder or dry ingredient blender allows you to make your own flours.
- An Instant Pot® facilitates large, one-pot meals that may be ideal for large families or planning meals for the week.
- A food processor helps with getting those six vegetables in at dinner. Ha! That step is coming.

Step 4: Be creative in the kitchen. Have fun! Real food doesn't have to be boring, and if the family (including children) are involved in the cooking process, they will be more likely to eat the food. Here are some ideas to involve the family in the cooking routine.

- Put on some music or a podcast during meal prep.
- Invite family members to participate. Be prepared for a possible mess if children are involved.

- Smell the spices and herbs.
- Taste-test along the way and decide together what should be added next. Encourage children to nibble on cut-up vegetables or other ingredients while helping, and let them watch you nibble, too.
- Buy special aprons that family members enjoy wearing during cooking.
- Try a new recipe. Put on a cooking show to get ideas.
- Grow some herbs in the kitchen or on your patio. Or create a garden outside, then add foods from your garden into your meals.
- Make homemade salad dressings, colorful yummy soups—create . . . and share!

Step 5: Commit to 30 days of REID. Thirty consecutive days of any new routine, whether it's to say hello to everybody you meet or exercise every day, is enough to change an action into a habit. What is critical, though, is that your 30-day commitment is to the full REID program. You may not see a benefit if you are still eating some processed or inflammatory foods.

Here are ways to encourage the entire family to participate in the new food lifestyle:

- For the three-year-old, eating a nutrient-rich meal enables the child to do some of their favorite activities afterward.
- If children don't understand the long-term reward system, a common strategy is to serve food in the order of nutritional benefit, so that they eat their favorite foods after consuming least favorite foods, which may be the vegetables. If that doesn't work, combine foods that are macronutrient balanced with fiber, protein, carb, and fat. For example, potatoes and carrots can be mixed with broccoli, kale, and ground roasted sunflower seeds, to which you can add cumin, garlic, and ginger. Don't forget fresh culinary herbs!
- For the adolescents and teenagers, you may need more incentivizing. One idea is to set up a special reward if they cooperate with the 30 days of REID plan. This could include a weekend camping adventure or special day trip with friends.

- To encourage family participation, discuss as a family a special family trip, vacation, or other activity as a reward for cooperating with the 30-day plan.
- Establish the understanding (especially with adolescents and teenagers) that this program of healthy eating doesn't go away after 30 days. What it does do is establish a solid foundation for a healthy lifestyle. After 30 days, family members can evaluate and discuss how they are feeling, and what effects they attribute to the new food lifestyle. Some teens may be reluctant to participate—I understand that. In that case, all you may be able to do is bring quality food into the house and let them choose. Buy the food you know is healthy, then prepare and serve it. If there is little else in the house to eat, they will eat what you make.
- Don't forget your pets! Yes, of course, many pet foods contain added glutamate and can be even worse than foods for humans.[1]

Be mindful that you and your family are worth the effort. Over a lifetime, we spend much more energy working every day to pay our bills and planning for a secure financial future than we spend on advancing our daily health. Yet, the best financial investment for our future may be what we eat now. Think about it: healthier seniors spend less on medical care. Not just our quality of life today but how healthy we are as we age will depend on what we decide at this moment.

The financial consequences of poor health should not be underestimated. I often think of how much money we saved when Taylor no longer required specialized home care, healthcare, and therapy treatments. Yes, the food we buy is expensive, but it is nothing compared to the cost of caring for a child with special needs. For many of my clients, their child's special needs are manageable only when one parent stays home with the child. The cost of that decision is the loss of one person's income. But we saved more than money when Taylor's symptoms were managed with our food choices. The time, energy, and stress we saved the family was priceless. My gratitude for the quality of life now afforded our family by these efforts is too emotional to put into words.

Goal 2: Eliminate Wheat Gluten and Processed Grains

Wheat and processed grains contain naturally high amounts of glutamate, as well as protein fragments that break down and release glutamate early in the digestive process. Remember, gluten in wheat was the original source of manufactured MSG.

Step 1: Replace wheat with unprocessed whole grains or other whole food carbohydrates. Purchasing whole grains avoids ingesting free glutamate and other byproducts that form during manufacturing processes, which include acid hydrolysis, fermentation, and defatting. The amount of free glutamate increases when you start to see on product labels ingredients that indicate processing, such as brown rice syrup, rice bran, parboiled anything, and even white rice. (Note that most white rice is made by removing the nutritious germ layer with a chemical process.) Some examples of whole grains with which to stock your kitchen include buckwheat groats, whole grain wild, black, red, or brown rice, quinoa, oat groats, and amaranth. Avoid the trap of replacing commercially processed gluten products with commercially processed gluten-free products. Some examples of food items to avoid are commercial cereals, gluten-free breads/pastries, grain crackers, and grain snacks.

Step 2: Replace commercial bread. There is no such thing as a "whole grain" bread if yeast or bacteria have been added. That is because, to make bread rise, yeast and bacteria ferment the grain. Once a grain is fermented and baked, the food belongs in the refined carbohydrate category. Flatbreads or homemade unleavened breads are good replacements for the common yeast or sourdough cultures used to leaven dough, cultures that add to bread's addictive properties.

Step 3: Use non-grain flours. Flour need not be from grains. Grinding seeds, nuts, roots, as well as whole grains, provides ample opportunities to incorporate variety in your crackers, flatbreads, waffles, muffins, or other baked goods. Making your own flours ensures you have control over the processing and storage. You can purchase whole grains like buckwheat groats and easily make your own flour with a simple coffee grinder or Vitamix dry blend container. Flours can be stored in mason jars in the fridge. Making your own flour as you need it avoids the chance of oxidation that can occur with commercial flours, and the potential for mold, which can be highly inflammatory. Also, you can blend any combination of nuts, seeds, and whole grains to make a wide variety of tasty gluten-free flours. Corn is also a grain and, again, if you eat it, source unprocessed products like organic corn on the cob.

Goal 3: Eliminate Dairy

There is a lot to be said on this topic, and here I want to break out some responses to frequent questions and concerns.

- First of all, why remove dairy? The major protein in milk and cheese is casein, which contains an exceptionally large amount of glutamate. When milk is pasteurized, homogenized, defatted, or further processed into cheese, casein proteins break down into free glutamate or glutamate-containing shorter peptides that are digested quickly in the upper gastrointestinal tract. Dairy products are usually placed in the highly processed food category.
- How do I get calcium without dairy? Replacing dairy with various nuts and seeds as well as adding a variety of green leafy vegetables and herbs will allow a diet with plenty of calcium. For many people, dairy is actually net *negative* on calcium. After consuming cheese, for example, the blood pH can drop. This triggers calcium to leach from your bones, as the body uses calcium from bone to maintain optimal blood pH. If your body becomes inflamed with dairy, there is even more leaching of calcium because inflammation also typically results in a lowering of blood pH.
- I love cheese and ice cream. What can I use as substitutes? In appendix B you'll find recipes for cheese substitutes (noncommercial) and homemade ice cream. More on substitutes in the next section. On a personal note, removing dairy was a game changer for me, and our family likes the substitutes.

Now that you have heard the arguments for *why*, this is *how* you eliminate dairy from your diet.

Step 1: Identify all dairy products and eliminate. This includes milks, yogurts, cheeses, and all the dairy byproducts in foods. Even "raw" cheese generally still falls under the category of highly processed dairy, unless you are making your own or live in a country that doesn't require 60-day aging and/or pasteurization of the final cheese product. I advise my clients to cut out all dairy initially. Once you have implemented the REID lifestyle and have reduced inflammation and improved your health, you can slowly try to introduce a less processed dairy product like homemade yogurt and see how it affects you.

Step 2: Avoid replacing dairy with convenient alternatives or tasty traps that are enriched with glutamate, such as many commercial non-dairy milks. There are a couple of commercial non-dairy milk products that only add nuts and water, but most add processed ingredients, and in the United States, all commercial non-dairy milks are pasteurized. Note that a common item in the vegan diet are nut cheeses. Avoid commercial nut cheeses, which are created with fermented nuts and are pasteurized. Fermentation and pasteurization help create that signature savory flavor—and an abundance of free glutamate. Make your own nut cheeses using the recipe in appendix B.

Also avoid non-dairy cheese replacements like Daiya® cheese or fermented legume products. Again, these products add a significant amount of glutamate to your diet.

Step 3: Replace dairy with your own savory recipes. Homemade nut and seed milks are a good replacement for animal milks. If you have a small child (over the age of one year) who is still consuming milk in a bottle, check out transitioning to nut and seed milks, as this may help with weaning from a bottle. Milk has a lot of sugar (lactose), which is one possible reason why children like it.

Nut and seed sauces add savory protein and fat to those plates of vegetables that will soon become routine. Avoid getting savory flavors through soy sauces, coconut amino acids, fish sauce, tomato pastes, or Braggs® amino acids, as these products also contain free glutamate from processing of proteins.

Goal 4: Increase Consumption of High-Fiber Vegetables and Herbs throughout the Day

You can eat unlimited amounts of these foods in the diet. There are very few things for which you can say that!

The variety of food choices in the produce aisle of a well-stocked market in the United States today is truly astonishing. The challenge is to introduce yourself to selections that may be unfamiliar. See table B.2, "Eat Your Veggies (A to Z)" in appendix B, and use this as your crib sheet to get started. Pick one to two new vegetables a week and incorporate them into your routine.

Also, a shout-out to more greens from grasses such as wheat grass (grass does not contain gluten proteins), oat grass, barley grass, alfalfa grass and, of course herbs: basil, bay leaf, cilantro, curry leaf, parsley, dill, lemon balm, oregano, sage, mint, rosemary, thyme, tarragon, marjoram, stevia leaves . . . the list goes on.

Often when I am working with families to help improve their food lifestyle, I encounter parents who state their child will not eat vegetables, or that their child will only eat foods like macaroni and cheese, and pizza. We were in a similar situation with Taylor; her diet was limited to industrially processed foods, which (frustratingly) we knew were devoid of nutrients. Despite our efforts to encourage her to eat her vegetables, she refused . . . to put it mildly. She would throw a tantrum at the sight of anything green on her plate.

The nutrient-void diet must be viewed as part of the health problem. Our bodies require various nutrients to thrive. Our nutrient requirements actually increase when we're combating inflammation. Optimal brain function also requires a variety of nutrients, and this is obtained through a variety of foods. With children or adults who are only consuming low-nutrient foods, I offer this perspective. We have a choice in what we feed our family and ourselves. We can continue to feed the addictions and pacify the persistent cravings, or we can break the addiction cycle and open up our palates to real, nutrient-rich food.

From microbial to human metabolism, we need to acquire our nutrients, in the right amounts and proportions, from whole foods.

Step 1: Here are some small steps to help transition the diet to more vegetables.

- Eat at least one green vegetable at each meal, including snacks.
- Serve at least three vegetables with every dinner (if you already consume three, try five, then six).
- Add three new vegetables per week to your routine.
- Use five vegetables in each smoothie batch, and add herbs.

Which brings us to smoothies. Smoothies are a simple and effective way to get the entire family to eat more vegetables, so let's go there.

Step 2: Learn to make smoothies. This is so important that I have created a video to show you how.[2] Smoothies are a great way to consume a full complement of a variety of nutritious raw vegetables, herbs, and other nutrient-rich foods all at once. It is particularly effective in adding the dark leafy greens to the diet. I now eat more leafy greens in one morning smoothie than I used to have in an entire week! Many children (including Taylor before we started smoothies) consume no dark green leafy vegetables at all.

Mixing ingredients like seeds, nuts, dates, beets, and kale stems requires a high-powered blending machine. Food texture is an important characteristic that drives our food preferences, and a blender with enough power to create a smooth consistency (thus the name smoothie) is essential. I've worked with many people, helping them change their food lifestyle and, hands down, Vitamix® is the preferred kitchen accessory for making smoothies. Nutribullet® is second.

The bulk of ingredients in a basic smoothie are raw organic vegetables and herbs. Other ingredients include seeds, nuts, and fruits. Place ingredients in the blender, add water to desired texture, include ice if desired, and hit start. That's it.

Appendix B provides some basic smoothie recipes. Here are some tips:

- Don't forget to add raw and organic nuts and seeds. These foods add proteins, fats, and various minerals to the smoothie—without protein powders.

- Remember, peanuts are not a nut, but a legume and are not advised for smoothies.
- Watch out for too much fruit in the smoothie. A smoothie consisting of mostly fruit, while more appealing to children, defeats the purpose of the smoothie, which is to increase the consumption of foods that are otherwise hard to get enough of in the diet.
- Add a rainbow of colors in your choice of vegetables, herbs, and fruits. These colors represent different micronutrients, like polyphenols and flavonoids, which are fantastic fuels for all our cells, human and microbial.
- Take advantage of seasonal and local farm-fresh foods.
- Don't forget the greens on the top of root vegetables like beets, carrots, radishes, rutabagas, and turnips. They are good, too!
- Waste not, want not. Use all parts of fruits and vegetables even if not typically considered the desirable portion. For example, use leaves from cauliflower, seeds and their hulls from squashes, tough stalks from broccoli, fennel, rhubarb, the skin of kiwi, and the husk of pomegranate, all of which contain many nutrients. After dinner prep, save the "undesirable" portions of foods for your smoothies.
- There are many edible parts of plants like flowers, roots, barks, leaves, seeds, fruits, and stems. How many barks do you have in your diet? Add two this week, such as cinnamon and pine bark.
- If the color green turns off members of your family, disguise the green with the addition of other brightly colored foods, like purple cabbage, beets, berries, carrots, and turmeric.
- If your child still doesn't like the look, serve their smoothie in a stainless-steel cup with a straw.
- For younger children, serve in fun-colored, reusable storage pouches.
- Remember, positive rewards can go a long way in influencing children to accept smoothies as part of their eating routine.
- Ideally, consume smoothies fresh.
- Smoothies can also be stored in a glass jar with a lid, such as a mason jar. Add a layer of liquid on the top to reduce contact with air and prevent oxidation (browning). You can store smoothies in this way for a couple of days.

- You can also freeze. Some creative families have poured smoothies into ice cube trays to ease the morning routine—at the touch of a button, you have an instant icy slurry. You can also serve frozen smoothies in the form of a popsicle during hot summer months.
- Avoid adding yogurts, non-dairy milks, honey, and agave.
- Rather than adding non-dairy milks, which have had the fiber removed, just add whole seeds, nuts, and water. This gives you the flavor of nut/seed milk, with the fiber. It's much easier, less wasteful, and less expensive, too.
- Most protein powders are processed and should not be used; nuts and seeds provide all the protein, fiber, and fats you need.
- Frozen fruits, vegetables, and herbs are fine to use.
- If new to vegetable smoothies, start out with 6-ounce portions (3 ounces for children under five) and work your way up to a filling amount every day. I consume about 12–16 ounces/day.
- Sometimes smoothies can have such a great effect on cellular metabolism (both human and microbial) that the body needs time to adjust. Some people may experience nausea for a couple of days, which is why I advise introducing your smoothie routine slowly.
- If your child refuses smoothies, start with homemade juice and slowly add in vegetable purees.

I can unequivocally say that I witnessed the effects of better food choices when I began my smoothie routine. I never ate so many vegetables before my smoothie routine became . . . well, routine.

Almost every client I have worked with, who stuck with the smoothies, reported feeling much better, even if they felt sick the first couple of days (detoxification). Results include greater energy, fewer moods swings (from spikes in carbohydrates and sugar), less sugar and carbohydrate cravings, and improved digestion. Even clients who struggled with high blood pressure reported reducing or going off blood pressure medication (see your doctor before altering any medication). The increased fiber is enough to make most people have very regular bowel movements.

Step 3: Sneak Attack. If smoothies aren't for you or your family, everyone can still consume a variety of vegetables and herbs every day, some in their raw state. But it takes planning! Be creative and sneak in the vegetables, even if you must be sly. Snacks like homemade kale chips, or dips with greens like cilantro, basil, and spinach, can add to the family's total consumption of vegetables, particularly leafy green vegetables.

Here are some of what I call Sneak Attack ideas:

- Dress up vegetables by topping with nut or seed sauces; these go particularly well with broccoli and cabbage.
- To sauces like curry or marinara, remove from heat after cooking and add pureed raw vegetables.
- Add raw chopped or pureed greens to different kinds of soups. The way to do this: cook the soup as desired. Pour hot soup into a bowl and, as it cools, add some raw chopped or pureed green leafy vegetables.
- Add pureed veggies to various dips or spreads, like pesto, hummus, black bean dip, guacamole, and pâtés.
- Add a variety of shredded vegetables to meat loaf, bean patties, frittatas, scrambled eggs, muffins, tacos, and more.
- On hot days, make popsicles with pureed vegetables.
- To waffle or pancake batter, add beets, squash, carrots, kale, and herbs such as cinnamon, nutmeg, cardamom, and cloves.
- To salads (a quinoa salad would be perfect) add finely chopped broccoli, cauliflower, and shredded cabbage, beets, rutabaga, and carrots. Alternatively, puree the vegetables and make a tasty dressing from them if you require a more covert operation.
- Chop various vegetables very small so a child can't pick out the pieces.

In my experience, I have found that the most desperate time for food is right before dinner. The aroma of the food cooking and the time of the day typically cause people to start gathering in the kitchen, rummaging for food. The risk here is family members grabbing a bunch of nutrient-poor snacks and ruining their dinner. Don't let your plans collapse; instead, take advantage of your family's appetite. Put out an assortment of cut vegetables, with perhaps a dip, ready for munching.

This is a great way to get the family to consume vegetables even before sitting down for dinner. Some pre-dinner snack ideas include:

- raw green beans, peppers, broccoli, and cauliflower with hummus or tahini dip
- carrots, jicama, and cucumbers with guacamole
- snap peas, kale chips, beet sticks, rutabaga chips
- roasted asparagus dipped in oil with lemon and garlic
- broccoli or cauliflower with pesto or a veggie/herb paste
- green salad
- shredded veggie slaw

Limiting snacking right before dinner to healthy foods will help increase the amount of nutrients in the diet overall. And remember: hunger is the best sauce.

You should know that shelled peas, potatoes, and yams are starchy vegetables, not high-fiber vegetables. The composition of these foods is better defined as a carbohydrate and should be considered a starch serving and not a vegetable serving. While some lettuces have good fiber, they're not as rich in nutrients as dark green leafy vegetables like collard greens, chards, kale, dandelion greens, mustard greens, and beet greens.

Goal 5: Clean Out Your Environment (Start with the Kitchen)

Now that you and your family are eating differently, it's time to clean house. Staying disciplined on the food journey is easier if the kitchen is filled with organic, whole food ingredients. This generally means cleaning many food items out of your cupboards and refrigerator.

Step 1: Review the list of ingredients that contain glutamate or its analogs in table 2.2 in chapter 2, and then review food products in your kitchen. Once you go through your pantry and refrigerator, you'll realize that most commercial condiments, sauces, dressings, dips, pre-made snack foods, seasoning packages, cereals, and nearly all packaged foods have ingredients that contain free glutamate, in addition to other processed ingredients that do not belong in your body. Removing commercially processed foods from your pantry goes a long way toward removing inflammatory additives from the food you feed your family. Eating whole foods is simpler and healthiest.

Step 2: Be careful about incorporating fermented foods into your whole food diet. While a variety of fermented foods are increasing in popularity due to the perception that they are a source of beneficial probiotics and support health, a word of caution. Here are some tips about fermented foods.

- Ideally, the microbes in probiotic sources are already "trained" on fermenting fiber-rich foods like vegetables and herbs and have turned on the genes needed to digest vegetable fiber. Good examples are fermented foods like sauerkraut, kimchi without added sugars, and beet kvass. These probiotic sources contain microbes that can get right to work digesting vegetable fiber in the large intestine—they are ready to be members of a healthy microbial ecosystem.

- Avoid ferments involving foods in which most of the macronutrients are simple carbohydrates, refined sugars, protein, or fats. Examples include cheese, natto (fermented beans), kombucha, and dosas (fermented rice and lentils). These are examples of common fermented foods that contain glutamate and other inflammatory byproducts (alcohol, aldehydes, phenols, amines, etc.) created during the fermentation process.

Goal 6: Restock Your Kitchen

Quality control starts with what you bring home. If you stop buying addictive foods, then you won't find these foods in the house in those weak moments when you are tempted. This is your best chance to really feel a difference. Here are foods to restock the kitchen, and how to go about it.

Step 1: Identify the best food sources in your area, such as farmers' markets, natural food stores carrying local produce, local farmers and hunters, your own farm. If you live near the coast, check out what fresh fish or other seafood is available daily on the docks. Get to know where your food comes from. No need to read a label to know what you are eating when it's whole food from the ground!

Step 2: Consult the list of ingredients to avoid, found in table 2.2, and take that list to the supermarket. Give yourself ample time to read labels and familiarize yourself with whole food items. Scrutinize every food that comes in a package. Ideally, do not take young children to the store the first few trips until you better understand how to translate what you read on food labels into foods to avoid. Then teach children what they can eat. Note that typically, whole foods are placed in the outer perimeter of the grocery aisles. Plan ahead where you will take your grocery cart so that when you shop with young children, you can control what food they see.

Step 3: Load up! The bulk—working toward all—of the items in your grocery cart should be whole foods:

- Vegetables
- Fresh herbs/spices
- Nuts/seeds
- Meats/eggs (in moderation); pasture-raised/grass-fed, wild-caught—animals subsisting on natural diets. Buy fresh and avoid cured meats or meats that contain rubs and preservatives (e.g., bacon, ham, prosciutto, sausage, pepperoni, prepackaged meats).
- Fruits (in moderation)
- Legumes (lentils and beans) (in moderation). Buy dry and prepare them yourself. Avoid cans.
- Whole grains (in moderation); quinoa, long-grain rice, coarse-ground corn (may need to avoid at first), buckwheat groats, oat groats, amaranth.
- If possible, buy only organic, with meats being both organic and grass-fed/pasture-raised or wild-caught.
- In general, avoid GMO (genetically modified organism) foods. This is because of the potential for them to be contaminated with chemicals such as glyphosate, the active ingredient in the herbicide Roundup®.
- If in doubt, don't buy it. Ingredient labels do not tell the whole story; the big unknowns are the manufacturing processes and harvesting practices that are not transparent to the consumer.

- Switch to natural sweeteners like whole fruits, stevia leaves, licorice root, raw organic honey. I use fruit to sweeten foods that need sweetening—dates can be used to make a great syrup.
- Plan out a few days of meals and stock up on pantry basics like oils, herbs, spices, nuts, seeds, beans, lentils, and whole grains. For meal plans, see appendix B.

A note on oils: oils have different *smoking points*, which is the temperature at which an oil starts to smoke. At this temperature, oils oxidize and create free radicals, which cause inflammation in the body. Use oil that won't smoke at the desired cooking temperature. Also, store oils in a dark, cool place because oils oxidize faster when exposed to sunlight and elevated temperatures. The use of canola, sunflower, safflower, vegetable, corn, and other inflammatory oils should be eliminated or extremely limited due to their poor omega-6/omega-3 fatty acid ratios, potential glyphosate exposure, and inherent inflammatory properties.

- Olive oil is good for dressings, dips, spreads, and sauces. It has a low smoking point and therefore avoid for high- and medium-temperature skillet cooking. Standard baking temperatures are fine, but avoid olive oil when broiling.
- Avocado and walnut oils have a high smoking point and are good for skillet cooking. These oils are produced with less processing than oils from seeds.
- Coconut oil has a medium smoking point and is good for low- to medium-temperature cooking. Avoid using coconut oil in stir-fry or high temperature cooking.
- Ghee (clarified butter) or fat trimmed from meat cuts is also fine, to add oil variety.

A note on spices and herbs: When available, use fresh spices and herbs, which are more potent than dried. However, many herbs can't be sourced fresh and the next best thing is dried. Note that dried herbs and spices oxidize and lose the potency over time, so they are best if you buy them in their biggest "whole" form, such as whole cloves, cinnamon sticks, sprigs of thyme, rosemary needles, and whole nutmeg, and then grind them before use. In this form, the oxidation rate is slower than if they are ground fine and then stored. Ground herbs are best if used or replaced every three months.

Things to keep in mind when sourcing herbs and spices:

- Organic or wildcrafted herbs and spices are best.
- Avoid vague ingredient labels like "spice blend," "spices," "proprietary spice blend."
- Avoid additives in spices like silicon dioxide or anti-caking agents.
- Avoid commercial "powders" like onion powder and garlic powder. These products are often irradiated or fumigated, heated, and flow agents added to prevent caking and sticking to manufacturing equipment. Use fresh—fresh garlic and onion have so many great health benefits!

Know your food sources: Investigate your foods. The savvy consumer is always on this journey, aware of the ever-changing landscape of what's going on in the food supply. In the following list of things to consider, the healthiest choices are in **bold**.

- Farm animals:
  - How were they raised? (cage, cramped, industrial, or **small-scale**)
  - How were they fed? (grains, organic grains, **pasture-raised, grass-fed**)
  - Were they given antibiotics as standard practice? (yes, **no**)
- Freshwater fish and seafoods:
  - Where did it come from? (imported, **local**)
  - How was it raised? (farmed, **wild-caught**)
  - How was it stored? (**fresh, fresh-frozen**, previously frozen/thawed)
- Farming practices:
  - Where is the farm located? (**local, rural**, within the country, foreign)
  - How is the soil rated? (**organic, wild-crafted** [**herbs**], conventional)
  - What is grown on the farm? (few crops, **variety of crops, crops rotated**)
  - What is the farm size? (industrial, **small, diverse, family farm**)

While you will not get answers to all these questions from your neighborhood grocer, asking these questions within your community can help you organize your approach to food sourcing. In the end, it may come down to making compromises. The point is to start investigating where your food comes from, and not walk away from the grocery store empty-handed because nothing is "good enough." Just keep in mind that it is only when you *think* about what you are buying can you choose the best of what is available in your area, and what fits your budget.

Goal 7: Eliminate Refined Sugars and Reserve Fruit as a Treat

Getting rid of refined sugar in your diet is critical for balancing your energy needs and reducing inflammation. Beet and cane sugar are both refined sugars. Note that, like glutamate, sugars have over 50 different names in commercially processed food products. Other names for sugar include sucrose, glucose, fructose, lactose, maltose, dextrose, and maltodextrin. Syrups (such as corn, rice, and maple syrup), fruit concentrates, fruit or chocolate liquors, and malts are some other sources for sugars. Even sugars naturally found in fruit should be consumed in balance with other nutrients.

The good news is you can eliminate many of the sources of refined sugars by eliminating commercially processed foods. Even items that are savory or spicy can have significant refined sugars added. The same is true for salad dressings, sauces, and dips. Baked goods, cereals, and commercial pancake and waffle mixes top the "Avoid" list, as they generally have added sugars, along with many additives, and are highly processed. The truth is, many of us consume a breakfast that more resembles a dessert in terms of sugar and nutrient content. When you make your own *everything*, you can choose the purest of ingredients and truly make it about your health. When Taylor turned 12 years old, she asked if she could have a waffle that wasn't green for her birthday. I acquiesced. Yes, I regularly put vegetables in my batters—check out the waffle recipe in appendix B. One more thing: you may be asking, can I have some chocolate? A square of good quality dark chocolate is fine for most. Just don't eat the whole bar!

Here are some tips to reduce sugar in your diet:

- Sugar is sugar, even if it is from a whole food fruit. I've spoken with many parents who are thrilled about their child being on a whole food diet, but the children are eating 6 to 10 servings of fruit a day. Remember that fruits and vegetables are not interchangeable and should not be lumped together in recommended serving sizes. A variety of fruits is fantastic in the diet, but in moderation—like it's a treat, or perhaps a topping for a delicious chia seed pudding. For many, microbial imbalance is a significant problem, and having too much fruit in the diet may promote microbial overgrowth in the small intestine.
- Eliminate or reduce fruit juices. All commercial fruit juices should be eliminated, as the manufacturing process destroys nutrients and incorporates additives. Even homemade freshly squeezed fruit juice removes fiber and packs a sugar load close to the amount in a soda. Once you remove all refined sugars that are coming into the diet from other sources, simple, whole fresh fruit is a very satisfying sweet treat.
- Avoid or limit dried fruits, particularly commercial dried fruits. The fruit drying process often uses sulfates, which can be problematic for many who are experiencing microbial imbalance. When used in moderation, though, dried fruits are concentrated sources of sugar that can help satisfy sugar cravings and transition from sugar addiction.

Goal 8: Identify Your Go-To Foods

Our weakest moments are when we are hungry, when we become vulnerable to eating anything. Find out what works for snacks for the family and have these snacks readily available to combat those low-energy moments that make us reach for simple carbohydrates. Having a plan avoids the desperate feeling that excessive hunger brings on. Here are some tips.

- Have a backpack that contains snacks that you take with you on day trips. Examples of healthy snacks include homemade trail mix, homemade protein bars, fresh fruit, chopped vegetables and dip, homemade root vegetable chips (such as a beet, rutabaga, sweet potato, yam, and potato mix).

- Pack snacks in the car for emergencies. Homemade trail mix is good for this.
- Have ready-made items available when you are hungry, such as vegetables and dip, trail mix, chicken and vegetable salad, hard-boiled eggs, and sliced apples or pears topped with nut butter. Even a cup of soup from a big batch does the trick, particularly on a cold day.
- Have a low energy, no-time-to-make-dinner strategy ready as a back-up plan. Stock your freezer with homemade soups, stews, chili, bean and vegetable patties, waffles, and muffins to have quick options available. Have frozen vegetables available as a backup. Make up some protein bars and store some in the freezer for emergencies. Avoid the "hangry" response. *Hangry* is a term that describes people who are so hungry they become angry.

Planning meals on weekends or days off makes it much easier to have healthy food on hand throughout the week. This helps avoid the trap of relying on unhealthy convenience foods during busy work and school days, when we're inevitably strapped for time. Soups and casseroles, for example, can be made in advance, stored, and eaten throughout the week for evening meals, as well as lunches and snacks. A large batch of quinoa can be used throughout the week for salads or can be transformed to a main course by adding a medley of sautéed vegetables. One thing I do routinely is soak and cook legumes in big batches and store extras in the freezer to facilitate quick meal preparation. A batch of garbanzo beans can be used to whip up a vegetable hummus or becomes a hot meal with vegetables and tomato sauce.

Here's another tip: When you return from a farmers market or grocery store, if you take the time to wash, soak, dry, and store your produce, your produce will last longer and be easier to use throughout the week. Chop up vegetables for you and the family to snack on while dinner is being prepared.

Goal 9: Have a Quality Control Plan for Consuming Foods Outside the Home

Unfortunately, we are all bombarded with unhealthy food choices as soon as we go out into the world. The typical children's birthday party, for example, where almost everything served is processed—hot dogs, pizza, sugary drinks, cake, ice cream—can be a real problem. In the workplace, coworkers bring homemade baked goods or a box of doughnuts to share with colleagues. Employers trap you in lunch meetings and offer you nothing but processed foods. Drive for a few hours on a family road trip, and the only food available is fast food. How can we control the quality of what we eat when so much of the food offered is not real food? Answer: have a plan.

Social Events: Indeed, feeling included in social events can be challenging if much of the food served can make you unwell. Unfortunately, processed foods high in MSG have become the standard fare at many social events because of the convenience. One rule of thumb is to bring food (a favorite dish to share?) for any social event, like a kale-quinoa salad, even if it's just a backup. If you don't know what will be served, don't leave it to chance that there may be some food available to eat.

Birthday parties: Pack your child's food for the event. You can send your child off with homemade pizza and a slice of homemade orange almond cake, homemade cupcake, or nut butter cookie, and feel good that they can have fun without the MSG and sugar load. Fortunately, most birthday parties will have fun games and activities that allow children to play with friends, and most children will enjoy themselves without the birthday cake. Of course, it's challenging for a youngster to watch as all their friends eat a cake dripping with icing. However, kids can learn at an early age that eating healthy is one of their family's core values, and that it is important that they make good food choices.

Dinner parties—children welcome: If you know the host of the dinner party well and it's just your family or a small gathering, you can decide whether it's worth trying to steer the menu toward foods that your family can consume. Fortunately, there has been an uptick in dietary consciousness, and discussing dietary restrictions in advance of a social gathering is much more commonplace these days. You can offer to bring a dish to share and provide a few examples of other dishes that you find delicious and think the host might, too.

If giving the host suggestions for food is awkward, and I can think of a few times this happened to me, you can always fuel up before your visit, bring some food (particularly for the most sensitive in the family), or eat after you get home. People do this all the time. You don't have to explain yourself or justify the restraint you show at the table with a list of health concerns or the scientific rationale behind your new food lifestyle. The simple statement "I'm on a diet" is acceptable anywhere, can mean anything, and says everything.

Holiday gatherings: Whether a work event, school party, or family get-together, the larger the gathering, the more likely there won't be real food to eat. Plan ahead. The more satiated you arrive at these events, the less likely you will be tempted to deviate.

Children's school: I never imagined the challenges I would face protecting my children from unhealthy foods while they were at school. Early in Taylor's diet transition, when she had been at a special-needs school for four months, we eliminated gluten and casein from her diet. Despite all the media buzz about the GF/CF diet for children with autism, this school, with 25 percent of the class made up of children with autism, was surprisingly unsupportive of Taylor's diet. The school often blatantly disregarded our dietary preferences, which at this point was just GF/CF and not the healthier REID lifestyle we adhere to today. We found out about it only after Taylor was served an offending food. When I objected, one of the lead teachers at the school told me that I was wasting my time and causing Taylor to be excluded from social events. I'm often shocked at schools that are unwilling to support parents who object to their children being pumped with commercially processed foods.

The most vulnerable age for children at school is preschool. The children may be too young to advocate for themselves, and may even take their classmate's food. My advice if you have preschool-age kids: work with the school to determine how far they are willing to accommodate your child's foods. Be clear with a written request that you only want your child to eat the foods you bring from home. If the school is not willing to accommodate that request and cannot provide a safe environment for your child, this may not be the best school for your child. Work with your child's teacher to know when there will be food served to the class as part of festivities, and then provide your child with foods that enable them to participate. For example:

- Make a batch of cupcakes, dress with frosting and top them with a slice of fruit for school celebration events. They can easily be stored in an airtight glass or stainless steel container in the freezer for several months. Simply pull one out the morning of the event and let thaw at room temperature.
- Supply the teacher with a treat for your child to have on hand as a backup if there is an unplanned special event. This could be a homemade cookie, fruit popsicle (if the school has a freezer), even some raisins may work in a pinch.

At any age, children are inundated with terrible food options at and around school. As a community, we can influence how schools feed our children. I'm a big fan of "no food sharing" policies at schools.

It's important to feel that your family's values toward food are accommodated on school grounds, and it is worth the effort to ensure that happens. What I did was provide all the food and liquid my child needed for the day when under the supervision of others. Very few people are aware of the pervasive use of MSG in foods. Therefore, if you're serious about establishing a healthier diet for your family, do not trust anyone to prepare your food or feed your children unless they are very familiar with ingredient labels and food processing. Ideally, the school educates the children, and *you* feed them.

Workplace: Pack your lunch for work. Bring some snacks in case you get hungry. Sometimes a handful of carrot sticks with hummus is the perfect way to chomp away the frustrations of a day at the office. If you have a commute to work, bring snacks for times you are stuck in the car. This last tip makes for a happier commuter and a more pleasant person when arriving at work or returning home (compared with someone who is beside themselves with hunger). My favorite is my own trail mix and an apple for the commute.

- Make extra food for dinner to have leftovers for lunch.
- Stock up on food storage containers. Glass containers are good; stainless steel is a better option for young children, or if you are concerned about breakage.
- Pack a portion of your morning smoothie in a mason jar and take it with you to work.
- Store snack foods like nut butters, homemade trail mix, and flax crackers in work area drawers for emergencies.
- If you don't have time to pack your lunch, have your handy go-to snacks. Some ideas are raw vegetables, nuts, seeds, and fruit.
- Bring your own food to on-site lunch meetings unless your company can accommodate your food needs.
- Don't let your guard down during off-site business lunches or dinners. Order bland items that are less likely to be offending, like salad with just oil and salt for dressing, and meat without sauces. Inquire what the restaurant uses for spices in soups and other dishes when ingredients aren't transparent.

Travel and Vacations: The key to controlling food quality outside the home is to always have healthy food available, which means you might have to bring it. Plan for door-to-door food options during travel. Ensuring that your family consistently eats healthily means being prepared and cautious, and resisting temptation.

When you absolutely cannot help eating something you know should be avoided, mentally note the changes in yourself or your child. Use the experience as motivation to increase your efforts to eliminate these foods. Without reminding yourself why you are making the effort, it is very easy to get on the slippery slope, drifting so far off your food lifestyle that it just seems like too much work to get back on track. Of course, life happens: moving day, holidays, kitchen remodel, the arrival of new babies. . . . Welcome the opportunities that follow disruptive life events to resume your practice.

If you are traveling on your trip by car, here are some tips:

- Pack plenty of food for your trip, and even include snacks for when you arrive at your destination. Homemade trail mix, vegetables and dips, salads, fruits, casseroles, and even soups in a thermos are all good options.

- Bring your Vitamix with smoothie makings in a cooler. (This is great if you are in a hotel room with no kitchen.) Also, bring your crockpot or Instant Pot with a ready-made meal. This can be consumed during your travel, or reheated and enjoyed once you reach your destination.
- Scout places to stop to eat along the way. These could be tables inside a grocery store where you can eat your carefully selected store purchases, a suitable restaurant, or a nice scenic park to eat the food you brought.

With plane and train travel, there is limited space for carrying food or food prep equipment. Here are some tips for this type of travel:

- Pack enough food for the time you leave your home to a few hours after you plan on reaching your destination.
- Use containers to pack individual hearty meals for the travel if it is a long trip. Some examples are quinoa salad with various ingredients; vegetables, rice, and meat; hummus with falafel patties and vegetables; and bean patties with tahini.
- Keep snacks such as homemade trail mix, fruit, vegetables, and homemade protein bars handy during your travel.
- Pack foods in a suitcase for when you arrive. By the time you reach your destination, the family is often exhausted, and having some food options available immediately will buy you time while you figure out where you are going to eat.
- As with car travel, before you depart for your trip, research places near your destination for grocery shopping and possible restaurants for dining. In our family, we often choose our vacation destinations based on available healthy eating options.

Remember—figure out the food *before* you embark on your trip.

Restaurants: Often the biggest departures from our food lifestyle occur during extended travel when we must go to restaurants. No restaurant is going to report all the ingredients in their dishes—they don't have to. In fact, they are free to use labels such as "special sauce" or "secret recipe" in their meal descriptions.

I had a client call me once in a somewhat distressed state about his eight-year-old daughter Keli's behavior regression. He said, "We've been following REID, but she recently started behaving worse." I reviewed the food items in the diet. He told me that his daughter really liked chicken and they'd been having it often. After spending some time trying to sort out if food could be the source of the problem, I asked him where he was getting his chicken. He told me how much Keli just loved Kentucky Fried Chicken®. Mystery solved! KFC has one of the highest amounts of MSG in their food of any fast-food restaurant and that is the "Colonel's Secret Recipe."[3] I let him know that his daughter was craving that food because of the MSG. It's easy to make assumptions such as chicken is just chicken or fries are just fries, but many restaurants, particularly fast-food chains, intentionally add MSG to their food.

Most restaurants will claim that their food does not contain MSG and, for the most part, this may be the sincere belief of restaurant owners and chefs. Similarly, restaurant waitstaff almost always claim that their dishes contain no MSG when in fact most dishes contain significant amounts. Unfortunately, due to the lack of knowledge about ingredients and food manufacturing processes, you can't trust these assurances. I often take the opportunity to educate waitstaff by asking to see one of the spices used in their seasonings or salad dressings. It's easy to point out which ingredients contain MSG and free glutamate and serve up the 90-second version of this book. This information is sometimes not received enthusiastically. However, I find that most people I encounter are truly unaware of the many sources of glutamate in food, and most appreciate the information. And really, without taking advantage of such a teachable moment, how else *can* we improve our nation's health, one bite at a time?

Here's a story: Once while I was traveling, the hotel I was staying at offered a breakfast buffet. The first day I ate from the buffet, I chose potatoes and eggs. Almost immediately following breakfast I developed a wicked headache, which lasted the whole day. The next day, I didn't trust anything in the buffet and ordered eggs and potatoes with no seasonings from the menu. The waiter said, "We have that in the buffet and so much more for the same price." I told him that I could see that the potatoes clearly had some sort of spice on them and he replied, "The potatoes just have paprika and salt and that's it." I asked him if the paprika was pure paprika and he replied "Yes, it's just paprika." After telling him my concerns, I asked him if he wouldn't mind showing me the paprika container so that I could review the ingredient label. He was willing and returned with a paprika-colored substance in a large plastic container. The ingredient label contained at least twenty ingredients and the first ingredient was "monosodium glutamate." Ten other ingredients on the list contained significant levels of MSG, like "yeast extract" and "hydrolyzed soy protein." Paprika was about the fifth ingredient. I showed the waiter the ingredient label and explained that the seasoning in the container was really MSG with a small amount of paprika added for coloring. He was shocked and very appreciative of the awareness. There's no mystery why most people don't feel healthy while traveling. We have few alternatives to restaurant food!

Here are some tips for restaurant eating:

- Seek restaurants that market farm-to-table ingredients or local, organic, whole foods. Once you find your trusted local restaurants, ordering will become easier. I can't tell you how exciting it is to find a restaurant that prepares simple, whole foods without additives or secret ingredients.
- Some restaurant chains offer extensive salad bars, and these are worth checking out. They can be a lifesaver if you are on the road in an unfamiliar part of the country and know nothing about the area.
- When ordering from a menu, ask questions about how the restaurant prepares food and be sure to request no wheat, dairy, or soy. Ask how they prepare dressings, sauces, and even ask about their seasonings.
- If in doubt, order plain foods—meat without sauces, salads without dressing. Ask for a side of olive oil and lemon wedges to dress your salad.
- Bring your own herbs and spices, order foods without any seasonings, and then season to taste when the food is brought. After a few

weeks on this diet, you will find your own taste buds have awakened and you are much more attuned to the subtleties and flavors of fresh foods. Have fun with it!

Goal 10: Embrace the Journey toward the Perfect Plate

Everything you have done so far leads to this: delicious food that is healthy for you, healthy for the planet, and oh so good for your family. If I were to describe the perfect plate, I couldn't point to specific foods that make it perfect (too many!) but I could describe its characteristics.

Foremost, the perfect plate is *colorful*: it is red, yellow, purple, orange, and so many hues of green! Also, it has *textures*: it is crunchy, silky, crumbly, firm, and chewy. And it is *flavorful*: it is savory, tart, tangy, fruity, sweet, sour, spicy, and imbued with the natural umami flavor that comes from ripe, fresh fruits, vegetables, nuts and seeds.

Appendix B, "The Perfect Plate: Recipes, Ingredients, and Meal Plans," can get you started. You may feel that you are learning how to cook all over again. (Great! It's an adventure!) Rather than thinking of all the foods that will be eliminated or reduced in your diet, consider all the *new* foods you are adding. Challenge yourself to try new vegetables, herbs, and ferments. I remember bringing an unusual item from the produce aisle to the grocery checkout and having the clerk ask me, "what's this?" I said I didn't know, but I was going to learn how to cook it that night! It was celery root.

Grow your own food if you can. Consider all the parts of a plant that are edible, and find new appreciation of how your foods are meant to nourish. Do your best with the resources you have available. Explore various combinations of herbs to add different tastes to your foods. Try new recipes and create your own.

Nutritional Supplements

What about supplements? That's what I tried, at first. Recognizing that my daughter had a very limited diet, and not knowing better, I initially resorted to store-bought supplements to provide important nutrients. However, through my research I discovered that many nutritional supplements contain free glutamate, as well as many other additives such as glutamine, which is quickly converted to glutamate in the body. Here's a different approach. Often, for the cost of a one-month supply of common supplements, you can buy a Vitamix and replace the supplement routine with fresh whole foods. Let's look at the nutrients in a simple smoothie with just the six ingredients listed in table 8.1.

Table 8.1. A Simple Smoothie Recipe (This is delicious—try it tomorrow morning!)

¼ cup	hulled sunflower seeds
¼ cup (50 g)	butternut squash
¼ cup	blueberries
¼ cup	parsley
⅓ medium size	avocado
12 sprigs	cilantro
1 cup	water

Now see table 8.2 that lists the nutrients in just one cup of the smoothie.

All this with just six ingredients! And that's just a small part of REID.

Through my research and work with many clients, I have seen that the amount of free, readily absorbed vitamins and nutrients provided by commercial supplements can prove too much for the body's cells, which go into metabolic overdrive to process the nutrients. Worse, the ingestion of a sudden bolus of supplement coming too fast, too much, can result in the short-term buildup of the products of metabolic reactions, causing a toxic response. Such a chemical imbalance can, as you might expect, increase glutamate signaling. What's more, the easily digestible nutrients in supplements can encourage microbial activity in the small intestine—something that needs to be avoided, as it can increase inflammation and glutamate signaling as well.

Table 8.2. Nutrient Facts: Simple Smoothie (250 ml or approximately a cup)

Macronutrients		% RDA (average adult male)
Protein (g)	15.2	20%
Carbohydrate (including fiber) (g)	48	11%
Fat (g)	46.26	60%
Micronutrients		
Calcium (mg)	400	20%
Magnesium (mg)	169.5	48%
Potassium (mg)	1917	41%
Phosphorous (mg)	317	45%
Iron (mg)	4.45	44%
Vitamin K (mcg)	320.5	290%
Vitamin A (mcg)	7289	909%
Vitamin C (mg)	44.6	50%
Vitamin E (mg)	10.6	67%
Vitamin B1 (Thiamin) (mg)	0.307	28%
Vitamin B2 (Riboflavin)	0.22	20%
Vitamin B3 (Niacin) (mg)	4.65	31%
Vitamin B4 (Choline) (mg)	34.6	10%
Vitamin B5 (Pantothenic) (mg)	2.283	46%
Vitamin B6 (Pyridoxine) (mg)	0.484	37%
Vitamin B9 (Folate) (mcg)	125.3	31%
Vitamin B12 (mcg)	0	–
Iodine (mcg)	0	–
Zinc (mcg)	3.34	30%
Selenium (mcg)	6.975	13%
Copper (mg)	0.42	47%
Manganese (mg)	1.6	85%

When considering the needs of the entire human ecosystem, generally supplements are not the best way to acquire nutrients, although there are some exceptions. Try whole foods first, and then determine your personal need for supplements, if any. In table 8.3 I've listed the whole food sources of the most frequently recommended supplements.

Table 8.3. Whole Food Sources of Commonly Supplemented Nutrients

Nutrient	Food Sources
Acetyl L-carnitine (ALC)	Meats, and vegetarian sources: eggs, quinoa, fenugreek seed, chia seeds, avocado, steel-cut oats
Alpha lipoic acid (ALA)	Broccoli, spinach, collard greens, chard, and other green vegetables/herbs
Beta glucan	Steel cut oats, shitake and maitake mushrooms, buckwheat groats
BH4 (tetrahydrobiopterin)	Salmon, sardines, mackerel, lots of rainbow-colored vegetables such as green leafy, cruciferous, root vegetables, and squashes for folate, vitamin C, and other antioxidants
Calcium	Cashews, almonds, collard greens, kale, turnip greens
Carnitine	Red meat, chicken, fish, avocado
CoQ10 (ubiquinol)	Organ meat, fatty fish, broccoli, eggs, sesame seeds, olives
Helps with ubiquinol production in the body	Dark leafy greens, green vegetables, sunlight
Copper	Oysters (seafood), kale, mushrooms, nuts, seeds, legumes, avocado
Dimethyl glycine (DMG)	Quinoa, beets, spinach, lamb
Glutathione	Asparagus, avocado, spinach, okra, broccoli, tomato, carrot, grapefruit, lemon
Helps with glutathione production in the body	Broccoli, cauliflower, cabbage, brussels sprouts, garlic, spinach, beets, turmeric, cinnamon, cardamom, black cumin seeds
Iron	Legumes, sunflower seeds, dark leafy greens, broccoli, asparagus, steel-cut oats (and other whole grains), thyme, parsley, sesame seeds, fennel, turmeric, celery seeds, hemp seeds, red meats
Lithium	Legumes, mustard seed, pistachios, eggs, herbs, nightshade vegetables
Magnesium	Pumpkin seeds, dark green leafy vegetables, sesame seeds, cashews, salmon, mackerel, trout

Table 8.3. Whole Food Sources of Commonly Supplemented Nutrients (*cont'd*)

Nutrient	Food Sources
Quercetin	RAW—Chili peppers, asparagus, kale, berries, plums, peppers, onions, broccoli, sophora japonica leaf/flowers
Vitamin B1 (thiamine)	Salmon, flax seeds, whole grains, acorn squash, asparagus, mussels
Vitamin B2 (riboflavin)	Almonds, red meat, sesame seeds, oily fish (salmon, tuna), eggs
Vitamin B3 (niacin)	Mushrooms, avocados, whole grains, fish (tuna, salmon), sweet potatoes
Vitamin B6 (pyridoxine)	Various seeds, banana, apple, tuna, meats, broccoli, carrots, avocado, egg, various dark green leafy greens, cauliflower, berries
Vitamin B7 (biotin)	Egg, liver meat, salmon, sardines, almonds, avocado, sweet potato, cauliflower, mushrooms
Vitamin B9 (folate)	Leafy greens, asparagus, beets, brussels sprouts, broccoli, avocado, nuts/seeds, citrus fruits, beef liver
Vitamin B12	Fish (sardines), organ meat, eggs, fermented vegetables, muscle meat
Vitamin C	Beet, carrot, spinach, broccoli, kale, cabbage, parsley, brussels sprouts, ginger, cauliflower, cranberries, asparagus, acai berries, strawberry, cherry, blackberry, blueberry, raspberry
Vitamin D3	Sunlight (20 min/day), UVB lamp (requirement that some portion of UVB spectrum are wavelengths less than 300 nm). To a lesser extent, a source can be fatty fish (salmon, sardines, tuna, mackerel), egg yolks
Vitamin E	Almonds, sesame seeds, sunflower seeds, avocados, trout, and to a lesser extent green leafy vegetables and broccoli
Zinc	Oysters, pumpkin seeds, sunflower seeds, cashews, whole grain buckwheat

This is derived from my own experience working with a variety of medical and naturopathic doctors, and from the reporting of my clients who have been recommended supplements. Note that many foods are sources for more than one nutrient—as we should expect from a whole food.

Ideally, we look to *foods* to nourish our bodies, not supplements. This is because nutrients benefit us most when partnered with various cofactors found in whole foods, which are not present in manufactured supplements. This has been known since the 1950s and 1960s. It's not the vitamin A that is great in carrots—it's the carrot.

After reviewing many patents and supplement manufacturing processes, I discovered that commercially available supplements are highly processed. They contain ingredients such as extracts, flavorings, and flow agents such as magnesium stearate. They have added sugars (e.g., maltodextrin, syrups), gelatin, oils, and lecithin, the very ingredients REID recommends eliminating. In addition, there is a big gap in research on the effects of supplements on the microbiome. While there may be exceptions to the general rule of avoiding supplements, the upshot is that you don't want to throw the kitchen sink at your body in the form a multivitamin when, say, you only need vitamin B6. Our nutritional needs are better balanced with nutrients obtained by eating whole foods.

Final Thoughts

If there is one lesson to be learned, it is that our food choices can make a huge difference in the quality of our lives. I hope that, by sharing my journey and the desperate circumstances that drove me to seek an answer to my family's health crisis, I can help others who are faced with similar challenges. But looking beyond what happened in my home, and what is happening in your home, what I discovered through research and personal experimentation has broader significance. Industrialized societies are facing their own health crises on a scale unprecedented in history. The central role of glutamate in mental illness, addiction, obesity, chronic inflammation, immune disorders, and autism demands that researchers take a hard look at the health effects of the enormous increase of environmental glutamate in food and personal care products we are exposed to today. This means that if scientists truly want to study the effect of glutamate on disease in human subjects, they must be meticulous in eliminating external sources of glutamate in the environment—sources one would hardly suspect, if you hadn't read the patents and researched the manufacturing processes as I have. If you have eliminated excess glutamate by cleaning out your pantry and refrigerator, and have purged suspect products from the bathroom, you know that it's a difficult thing to do. But that is the only way researchers can conduct a glutamate-controlled experiment on human subjects, and that's why it's an expensive clinical study to conduct.

As a scientist, I know that my experience with my daughter, family, friends, and now almost 2000 personal clients doesn't *prove* anything. Properly designed clinical trials need to be funded and conducted. What these accounts do provide, however, is a large body of anecdotal evidence that the reduction of dietary glutamate has significant health benefits for many with chronic inflammatory conditions. In our case, we observed drastic improvements in autism symptoms. Everything I've researched regarding the role of glutamate dysregulation in disease and the connection to dietary MSG suggests that we are on the right track. Call it a gut feeling, but that is how I read the scientific literature.

As you travel your own food lifestyle journey, you will find out what works best for you and your family. I wish you success, and courage, because if you are facing a health crisis, you are already under a lot of stress. But you've got this! Just think about the REID protocols in their most general terms: eliminate processed foods, reduce or avoid wheat, dairy, and sugar, eat plenty of vegetables and herbs, sprinkle with some fruit, nuts, and seeds, and include some meats and fish, if you desire. However far you take it, embrace the journey.

Good health,
Katie

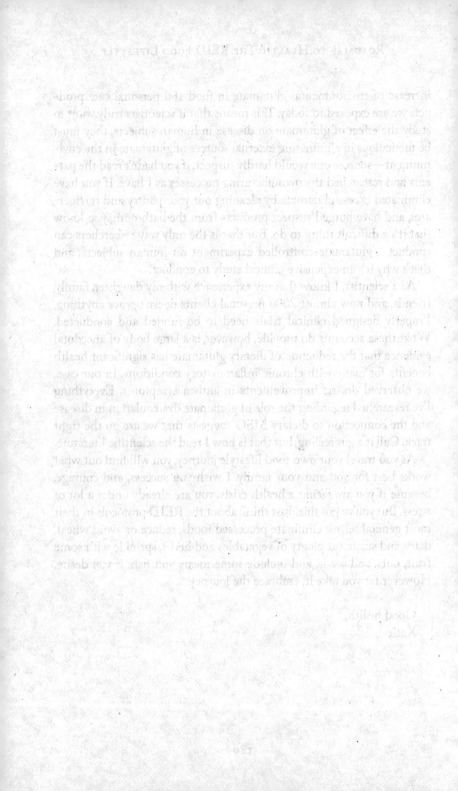

Appendix A

DO THE MATH: HIDDEN MSG
FROM PROTEIN IN PROCESSED FOOD

TO ESTIMATE THE TOTAL AMOUNT OF MSG IN NORTH AMERICAN
diets coming just from protein in processed food, I needed to know
how much processed food people ate, the amount of protein it contained, and how much of that protein is degraded during manufacturing. Fortunately, this information is available because scientists
interested in the impact of processed foods on human health have
studied how much of it we eat.[1]

In my calculations, I use the NOVA food classification[2] of factory-
processed food, the standard used in various studies examining the
diets of nations. NOVA classifies foods into four groups, based on the
nature and extent of processing. Table A.1 shows the NOVA groups
and some examples of foods in each group. Based on a Canadian study,
I am able to show approximately how much people eat from each
group, expressed as a percent of total calories ingested, given an average
consumption of 2064 kilocalories (kcal) per day.[3]

These data are consistent with other studies examining consumption of processed foods in other nations.[4] Note that the United States
is one of the greatest consumers of ultraprocessed food products in the
world.

This is how free glutamate from processed proteins was estimated in
each group. First, from the data in table A.1, I determined how many
kcal in each group comes from protein. Given that the average diet is

Table A.1. NOVA Food Groups and Percent of Calories Consumed Daily from Each

NOVA Food Group	Percent kcals* Consumed
Group 1: Unprocessed or minimally processed foods (e.g., vegetables, nuts, fish, uncured meats, juices, flours, pasta, yogurt)	39.2%
Group 2: Processed culinary ingredients (e.g., oils, salad dressings, powdered seasonings, syrups, ghee, butter, starches)	6.1%
Group 3: Processed foods (e.g., canned legumes and vegetables, breads, cheeses, cured meats, alcohol, and sauces)	7.0%
Group 4: Ultraprocessed foods (e.g., canned pasta, snacks, desserts, soda, instant soups, infant formula, energy replacement drinks, sweetened juices, frozen dinners, pizza, chicken nuggets, and over half of commercial breakfast cereals)	47.7%

*Note that the term kcal (kilocalories or 1000 calories) used by scientists is equivalent to the calories you would see on a food label. So, of course, the Canadians in the study (see note 3) are consuming only 2064 calories a day by those standards.

16.3 percent protein, if a person is consuming 2064 kilocalories per day, then 336 kilocalories of that is from protein.[5] Using the conversion factor of 1 gram of protein equals 4.1 kilocalories of energy, I am able to convert kilocalories of protein to grams of protein.

336 kcal/ day ÷ 4.1 kcal/g of protein = 82 grams of protein/day

Based on the degree of processing in each group, I then estimated the amount of free amino acids consumed. From there, I determined what percent of the free amino acids is glutamate.

Group 4

Let's start with the biggest contributor of MSG from processed proteins: ultraprocessed food. In their study, the Canadian researchers estimated that 8.5 percent of total kilocalories (175 kcals) in Group 4 foods comes from protein. Using the conversion factor of 4.1 kcal/g protein, we determine the grams of protein in Group 4 foods this way:

$$175 \text{ kcal} \div 4.1 \text{ kcal/g protein} = 42.7 \text{ grams of protein}$$

A conservative estimate is 20 percent of that protein by weight is glutamate. Because this group is ultraprocessed, the protein is nearly completely degraded, giving 8.5 grams of glutamate in free amino acids and hydrolyzed peptides.

Keep in mind, too, that 8.5 grams of free glutamate is a conservative estimate. Under acidic conditions used in many of the chemical manufacturing processes used to create Group 4 foods, the amino acid glutamine is converted to glutamate. Since *glutamine* has a similar abundance in proteins as does *glutamate*, the actual amount of glutamate in this category may be twice 8.5 grams. The conversion of glutamine to glutamate under acidic conditions is another example of how food processing increases the amount of MSG in food.

Group 3

On average, 7 percent of calories in the diet came from Group 3 processed foods, half of which (3.5 percent) was attributed to cheese alone. From cheese, 2064 kcal/day × 3.5% = 72 kcal/day. Cheese is made up of about 30 percent protein, so 72 kcal/day × 30% protein tells us that 22 kcal/day is coming from the protein just in cheese. Using the conversion factor relating kcals and grams of protein, we can calculate

$$22 \text{ kcal/day} \div 4.1 \text{ kcal/g of protein} =$$
$$5.4 \text{ grams/day of protein from cheese}$$

Recall that 25 percent of casein (the protein in cheese) is made up of glutamate. How much of this protein is degraded? The amount of protein degradation varies widely with the cheese manufacturing process.[6] The amount of enzymes and cultures added, and the time the cheese is allowed to age, are the largest contributors to protein degradation.

Conservatively, I'll estimate 50 percent of the protein is degraded in cheese (that is, 50 percent of the glutamic acid in cheese is either free amino acids or in small peptides). This means you can figure 5.4 grams protein × 50% protein degraded × 25% glutamate = 0.7 grams of glutamate is ingested each day, just from cheese the average person eats. And again this is an underestimate, as it doesn't account for glutamine in cheese that is hydrolyzed to glutamate during food manufacturing.

Additionally, from Group 3, approximately 2 percent of a person's total daily calorie consumption is coming from cured meats, meat substitutes, and processed nuts/seeds.[7] This amounts to 41 kcal/day. These are protein-rich foods, so I can assume approximately 30 percent of these calories are from protein. Thirty percent of 41 kcal/day is equal to 12.4 kcal/day. Converting to grams, that is equivalent to 3.0 grams of protein/day from this source. Now, these nut and meat proteins don't have to be excessively high in glutamate to add to the load, so conservatively, let's figure that only 10 percent of those grams come from glutamate and 50 percent of the protein is degraded. That's another 0.15 gram of free glutamate from the Group 3 food classification. Note that preservatives, flavors, and other additives containing glutamate are routinely added to Group 3 foods that are not counted in this estimate.

Breads are also in the Group 3 category. Bread is a staple in many diets, and is problematic because it is fermented, processed, and starts with a glutamate-rich protein, gluten. The amount of protein degradation in bread again depends on the manufacturing conditions. On average, I estimate 50 percent of the protein in bread is degraded, based on a review of manufacturing processes.[8] Researchers estimate that approximately 6 percent of total dietary protein intake comes from breads (this does not include cakes, pies, and gluten-containing desserts).[9] If 16.3 percent of calories in the diet are from protein, that is equivalent to 336 calories. If 6 percent of those calories is attributed to bread, that means approximately 20 kcal/day of protein is coming from bread. As before, kilocalories are converted to grams of protein using 4.1 kcal/g protein; this yields 20 kcal/day = 4.9 grams protein from bread. Approximately 50 percent of this protein (about 2.4 grams) is degraded, and 25 percent of that is glutamate, yielding 0.6 grams of free glutamate from bread.

From Group 3, adding together the contribution of cheese, breads, and processed meats only, the amount of free glutamate is estimated to be 0.7 g + 0.15 g + 0.6 g respectively for a conservative total approximation of 1.5 grams.

Group 2

Many of the processed culinary ingredients in Group 2 (e.g., salad dressings, powdered seasonings) contain free glutamate from processed proteins. Of the 2064 kilocalories consumed per day, the study shows that 6.1 percent of caloric intake, or 126 kcal/day, is derived from the foods in Group 2. Of this, approximately 25 percent is derived from protein. Calculating 25% × 126 kcal/day shows that 31.5 kcal/day come from protein in Group 2 foods. Converting kilocalories of protein to grams, we calculate 7.7 grams of protein from Group 2. Group 2 foods are less processed than those in Groups 3 and 4, and I'll estimate that only 10 percent of the protein is degraded, which gives us 0.8 percent free amino acids from protein degradation. Conservatively estimating that 10 percent of those free amino acids is glutamate gives us about 0.1 grams of free glutamate from Group 2.

Group 1

Group 1 contains minimally processed foods. This group sounds like mainly whole foods, but on closer examination, it's not entirely. Group 1 includes fresh or frozen meat, fresh or pasteurized milk and plain yogurt, whole or polished grains, fresh, frozen, or dried fruits, and unsweetened fruit juices. Standard manufacturing processes for Group 1 include cleaning and removal of inedible fractions, portioning, grating, flaking, drying, polishing, chilling, freezing, pasteurization, fermentation, fat reduction, vacuum and gas packing, squeezing, and simple wrapping. Group 1 also contains vitamin and mineral fortification to replace nutrients lost in processing. Ultrapasteurized foods, like the lactose-reduced milk you might drink, are also in this category. That's still a lot of processing going on. Even a conservative estimate would suggest that 10 percent of proteins obtained from Group 1 are degraded.

The calculation of free glutamate and/or hydrolyzed proteins coming from protein processing from Group 1 would then be as follows: the authors reported 37.7 percent of total calories is derived from Group 1. That is 778 kcal/day. Approximately 25 percent of these calories is from protein, which is 195 kilocalories. Using the conversion from kilocalories to grams of protein, 47.5 grams of protein (195 kcal/day protein ÷ 4.1 kcal/g of protein) is coming from Group 1. We assume conservatively that approximately 10 percent of this protein content is broken down to free amino acids or is at least partially hydrolyzed. Ten percent is equal to 4.8 grams. If 10 percent of that amount is free glutamate, that's another 0.5 grams of MSG being ingested from Group 1 foods.

Let's tally the amount of glutamate coming just from processed protein in the four groups:

Group 1: 0.5 grams
Group 2: 0.1 grams
Group 3: 1.5 grams
Group 4: 8.5 grams

This is the math used to populate table 2.3.

Appendix B

THE PERFECT PLATE:
RECIPES, INGREDIENTS, AND MEAL PLANS

USE THIS APPENDIX TO GUIDE YOU TO THAT PERFECT PLATE THAT feeds you, your family, and that vast population of microbes that is also "you."

Ingredients

Someone once told me that at any one time, the contents of a full refrigerator could be used to create a variety of delicious meals: a light lunch, a feast, late breakfast, romantic dinner for two. It was solely the cook's imagination—and the ability to select the necessary and reject those that were not needed—that determined the nature of the meal. In the same way, there is so much food available in modern societies, so to answer the question, "What do we eat?" we must first imagine what our meals *should* look like. Then, like the creative cook, we can select the ingredients that will lead us to health, and reject those that can make us unwell.

What to Eat, and What's a Serving?

Okay, now—what to eat, and how much of everything should we have every day? Table B.1 lists some recommended foods, and how much constitutes a serving. If some of these foods are unfamiliar, go online and you will find everything you want to know about them.

Table B.1. Food Serving Guidelines (based on 2000 cal/day)

Foods	Servings/day	Examples
High-fiber vegetables[a]	> 6 servings serving size = 1 C raw, ½ C cooked	kale, watercress, asparagus, broccoli, collard greens, chards, dandelion greens, beets with greens, carrots with green tops, artichokes, onions, cabbages, okra, mustard greens, rutabaga, squashes, fennel, brussels sprouts
Whole food proteins[b]	6–7 servings 1 serving = 1 oz meat, ¼ C cooked beans, 1 egg, 1 Tbsp nut butter, or ½ oz nuts or seeds	unprocessed meats, salmon, eggs, almonds, walnuts, pecans, chia seed, pumpkin seed, flaxseed, sesame seed, eggs, garbanzo beans, adzuki beans
Whole food carbohydrates	4 servings 1 serving = ⅓ C	starchy vegetables such as red potatoes, yams, sweet potatoes, turnips, jicama, cassava, rutabaga, Jerusalem artichokes, zucchini, butternut squash; whole grains such as steel-cut oats, oat groats, quinoa, wild rice (not white), red rice or black rice, buckwheat groats, amaranth; legumes such as lentils, beans; fruits (limit fruit to no more than two servings per day)
Fruits	1–3 servings 1 serving = ⅓ C fresh, 1 oz dry fruit	whole fruits (not juices): grapes, blueberries, strawberries, oranges, apples, kiwi, lemon, pomegranate, avocado, tomato, cucumber; avoid or limit high glycemic fruits like bananas, pineapple, and mangos
Whole food fats	2–3 servings 1 serving = 1 oz nuts or seeds, 1 small avocado, 1 oz fatty meat, or 1 Tbsp oil	olives, avocados, raw/unrefined oils (e.g., olive, avocado, coconut), seeds (sesame, chia, flaxseed, pumpkin), nuts (pecan, walnut, Brazil nut), nut butters, fatty meats (organ meat, fatty fish)

Table B.1. Food Serving Guidelines (based on 2000 cal/day) (*continued*)

Foods	Servings/day	Examples
Herbs and spices	unlimited to taste	variety, variety, variety: ginger, sage, peppermint, blackberry leaves, cinnamon, lemon balm, cloves, rosemary, oregano, cardamom, basil, cilantro, lemon grass, chamomile, turmeric, garlic, black pepper, cayenne, nutmeg, parsley, fenugreek seed, cumin seed, thyme, culinary sumac, marjoram, dill, mint, savory, tarragon, cayenne, bay leaf

[a] Ideally, consume 50% of vegetables raw. To retain the most fiber, cooked vegetables should be cooked lightly so still firm.

[b] Please review the discussion on how to source meat and fish in chapter 8. If possible, meat should come from animals fed a natural diet and raised in a natural environment. Fish should be wild-caught. Eat organic. Avoid processed meats such as lunch meat and any chicken that is cut up, breaded, and fried.

Meal Templates

Now, let's turn our whole foods into a meal. I plan meals by thinking in terms of *meal templates*, rather than specific recipes. The basic template balances energy sources and should contain some protein, carbohydrate, fat, and fiber (with the bulk of the fiber from vegetables). Add herbs (herbs are such amazing sources of nutrients that they sit at the apex of the REID food pyramid). This nutrient profile applies to every meal, including snacks. Of course, because nature does it best, some foods are power foods, containing multiple sources of energy. For example, an avocado is a non-sweet fruit containing healthy fat, carbohydrate, fiber, and even a small amount of protein. Sesame seeds contain healthy fat, fiber, and protein. How much to eat? Whether you have multiple servings of high-fiber vegetables at a meal, or rarely snack during the day, "how much" depends on factors like age, weight, and activity level. Follow your gut feeling about how much to eat.

To show you how this works, let's start the day with breakfast. First, identify your whole food protein. Today it is two eggs. Protein: √. Add a cup of assorted vegetables—raw, steamed, or sautéed. In this example we'll add broccoli, spinach, and cabbage. Vegetable fiber: √. For a carbohydrate, sauté a red potato with garlic in avocado oil. Carbohydrate: √. Fat: √. Sprinkle three herbs, such as rosemary, thyme, and oregano, on top of the potatoes. Herbs: √. Top with slices of avocado. Fiber: √. Fat: √. Carbohydrate: √.

Now, let's consider a dinner template. For dinner, select six fiber-rich vegetables—say, fennel, chard, beets, onion, celery root, and arugula. Now choose six herbs. Good choices are cumin, ginger, paprika, fenugreek seeds, coriander seeds, and turmeric. Add a starchy vegetable or whole grain such as quinoa. And top the whole thing with a protein- and fat-rich nut or seed sauce. Fiber, fat, protein, carbohydrate, herbs: √ √ √ √ √.

Weekly Meal Plan

Here is a sample of what a week of REID meals might look like. The perfect plate is many things, and every plate that is filled with a variety of fresh whole foods is perfect. Recipes for items with the asterisk (*) are at the end of this appendix.

Day 1

BREAKFAST: HOT OATS AND SMOOTHIE
6 oz smoothie*
⅓ C steel-cut oats (or millet seeds or buckwheat groats), cooked
Sprinkle on:
1 Tbsp flaxseeds
1 Tbsp ground sunflower seeds
¼ tsp each cinnamon and nutmeg
1 tsp turmeric
¼ C berries

SNACK: CRACKERS AND SPREAD

Seed crackers* and spread (i.e., chicken salad*, salmon salad, nut
    butter*, chutney, or bean dip)

LUNCH: CHICKEN AND BLACK BEAN–RICE SALAD

⅓ C wild black rice, cooked
2 oz chicken, baked or sautéed
2 C fresh chopped/shredded vegetables (e.g., spinach, mixed greens,
    kale, chards, parsley, carrots, cabbage, beets)
Top with nut sauce*

SNACK: FRUIT AND TOASTED NUTS OR SEEDS

¼ C fruit (e.g., ½ apple, ¼ C berries)
2 oz of slightly toasted nuts or seeds or nut butter*

DINNER: SALMON WITH BROWN RICE AND VEGGIES

3 oz grilled or baked salmon
⅓ C brown rice, cooked
Unlimited lightly sautéed veggies (try to add five or six for variety;
    e.g., broccoli, cabbage, beets, fennel, turnips, chard)
1 tsp olive oil
Top with chopped cucumber, tomato, avocado, parsley, cilantro, basil,
    dill, ground mustard (pick four items that sound good)

Day 2

BREAKFAST: EGGS AND VEGGIES

6 oz smoothie*
2 eggs (any style)
⅓ C sweet potatoes (baked or sautéed)
1 C sautéed spinach, peppers, tomatoes, onions
1 tsp turmeric, ginger, garlic (raw or sautéed)

SNACK: TRAIL MIX*

⅓ C trail mix

LUNCH: HOMEMADE YIROS (GYROS)
flatbread* or seed cracker*
2 oz of organic, grass-fed chicken (cooked, cubed)
⅓ C homemade nut cheese sauce*, with lemon, mustard, garlic, dill
½ C mixed chopped cucumber, tomato, onion
½ C mixed shredded cabbage, beets, carrots

SNACK: VEGETABLE CHIPS AND DIP
Assortment of thinly sliced vegetables (e.g., carrots, parsnips, beets,
    rutabaga, sunchokes, turnips, radishes, potatoes, sweet potatoes,
    cauliflower, kale, celery root) baked (300°F or 350°F) until crisp
    and dip (e.g., guacamole, hummus, tahini*, cauliflower dip*)

DINNER: ROAST MEAT AND VEGGIES
2 oz chicken or beef, roasted with 1 tsp olive oil
½ medium sweet potato, baked
2 C roasted vegetables (e.g., onions, beets, rutabaga, Brussels sprouts,
    peppers, broccoli, cauliflower, kale, garlic, sunchokes)
½ C lettuce greens (spring lettuce, arugula, spinach, radicchio)
Put uncooked greens on top of roasted meat and top with homemade
    nut cheese*, sauerkraut, or pickles

Day 3

BREAKFAST: SMOOTHIE WITH MUFFIN
6 oz smoothie*
1–2 Hearty Bite Muffins*

SNACK: HARD-BOILED EGG
1 hard-boiled egg (with salt or herbs)
10 carrot and fennel sticks with guacamole

LUNCH: CHICKEN SALAD*

SNACK: COOKIE AND CARROTS
1 homemade cookie*
carrot sticks

DINNER: CHICKEN AND VEGGIE STIR FRY*

Day 4

BREAKFAST: VEGGIE SCRAMBLE AND SMOOTHIE
6 oz smoothie*

2 eggs, scrambled

Add sautéed veggies and top with sliced avocado, chopped tomato and cilantro

SNACK: BERRIES AND GRANOLA
⅓ C mixed berries

⅓ C homemade grain-free granola*

LUNCH: VEGGIE COBB SALAD
1 C mixed leafy greens (e.g., kale, spinach, parsley, cilantro, chard, arugula)

1 hard-boiled egg

1 C roasted veggies (e.g., Brussels sprouts, squash, sweet potato)

1 C mixed chopped onions, cucumbers, tomatoes

2 Tbsp homemade tahini, lemon juice, and nut cheese dressing*

SNACK: NUTS/NUT BUTTER AND VEGGIE STICKS
Homemade protein bar*

Raw carrots and green beans

DINNER: WARM CHICKEN AND GRAIN SALAD
2–3 oz chicken or other meat

½ C cooked wild rice (or other grain like quinoa, buckwheat groats, millet)

2 C spinach and mixed greens

2 Tbsp homemade tahini, lemon juice and nut cheese dressing*

1 C raw veggies (e.g., shredded cabbage, cucumber, parsley, cilantro, broccoli, green beans, onion)

Day 5

BREAKFAST: WAFFLE AND SMOOTHIE
4 oz Veggie-licious smoothie*

1 veggie waffle* or pancakes with veggies*

Waffle toppings:
1 Tbsp date syrup*
⅓ C mixed berries

SNACK: AVOCADO AND FLATBREAD
⅓ avocado, sliced
flatbread square*
Top with chopped cilantro, tomato, and squeeze of lemon and salt
to taste

LUNCH: VEGETABLE FRITTER, SALMON, AND VEGGIES
3 oz cooked salmon
½ C finely chopped tomatoes, fennel and onions, cilantro, squeeze
of lemon
Combine ingredients into a salad and place on vegetable fritter*

SNACK: SWEET POTATO
½ medium sweet potato, cooked
Mix or mash potato with ground flaxseeds (or pumpkin, sesame,
sunflower seeds)
Top with ½ C chopped chard, pinch of cloves, black pepper, and
turmeric, 1 Tbsp coconut oil, and salt to taste.

**DINNER: HOMEMADE CHICKEN AND WILD RICE SOUP
WITH GREENS**
2 C homemade chicken and wild rice soup*
Place 1 C of uncooked chopped greens in bowl and into it ladle hot
soup. Suggestions for greens: cilantro, parsley, chards, mustard
greens, kale, arugula, mixed lettuce greens, spinach, dandelion greens

Day 6

BREAKFAST: PORRIDGE
1 C porridge*

SNACK: SMOOTHIE
6 oz Berry Fusion smoothie*

LUNCH: ZUCCHINI PASTA AND VEGGIES

1 C roasted spaghetti squash or spiralized zucchini or shredded beets
1 C marinara sauce*
1 C roasted vegetables (e.g., broccoli, brussels sprouts, mushrooms, cauliflower, beets)

SNACK: BOILED EGG AND VEGGIES

1 hard-boiled egg
green beans, carrot sticks, jicama
2 Tbsp tahini and mustard dressing* for dipping

DINNER: HOMEMADE FISH TACOS

2 tortillas* or crepes*
¼ C cabbage, shredded
¼ C beets, shredded
½ C black beans, cooked
3 oz cooked salmon or fish of choice
3–6 herbs (e.g., cayenne, cumin, ginger, black pepper, garlic, oregano, thyme)
Toppings: chopped onions, tomatoes, avocado, cilantro, sauerkraut, pickles

Day 7

BREAKFAST: SMOOTHIE

8 oz Veggie-licious smoothie*
½ C Apple Pear Crisp*

SNACK: VEGGIES AND NUT BUTTER

Flax crackers*
2 Tbsp homemade nut butter*
Mixed green beans, carrot sticks, cucumber slices

LUNCH: ROASTED VEGETABLE AND CHICKEN SALAD

1 C chicken salad*
½ C roasted vegetables of choice (or 1 C shredded raw rainbow vegetables)
Toss with 1 Tbsp lemon juice and 1 Tbsp tahini dressing*

SNACK: CRACKERS AND SARDINES
Flax crackers* with sardines
Green beans, fennel, parsnips, cucumber, carrots

DINNER: VEGETABLE CURRY*

Recipes

Here are the recipes for the week of meals described, plus some basic recipes that will come in handy when you start creating your own meals. For example, I use my pre-prepared nut butters, nut sauce, and tahini lavishly throughout the week, and you may, too.

Apple Pear Crisp

2 large apples, cored and chopped
2 large pears, cored and chopped
1 C nuts and seeds, chopped (e.g., pumpkin, sunflower, millet, flaxseeds, almonds, hazelnuts, Brazil nuts)
¼ cup unsweetened coconut flakes
2 Tbsp herbs (e.g., ground cinnamon, cloves, cardamom, nutmeg)
2 Tbsp melted coconut oil
Juice from half of a fresh lemon
2 Tbsp date syrup*
Pinch of sea salt

Preheat oven to 350°F. In a large bowl, combine the apples, pears, and lemon juice and mix. Place mixture on bottom of baking dish and bake for 10 minutes. In bowl, add chopped nuts, seeds, and herbs and mix. In a separate container, mix the coconut oil with the date syrup and pour over nuts and seeds and mix. Place this mixture on top of fruit in baking dish and bake for another 15–20 minutes until toasted. Let cool before eating.

Broth

For bone broth, source clean bones from animals fed their natural diet and raised in a natural environment. For vegetable broth, collect a variety of vegetable parts that may have not met the standard for serving, such as leek tops, ends of onions, kale stems, and cabbage cores. Add fennel, cauliflower, broccoli, bok choy, beets, rutabaga, radishes, or other veggies.

Place bones or vegetables in large pot and add 1 tsp each of a variety of herbs (e.g., rosemary, thyme, turmeric, cumin, bay leaves, fennel seeds, garlic). Add water to top of bones or vegetables. Bring to boil and simmer, covered, three hours or less. (Note: extending the cooking time for bones causes further breakdown of bone collagen, a protein, which increases the amount of free glutamate.) Cool broth sufficiently to handle and strain in a colander. Use immediately or store in mason jars in fridge for up to one week or freeze for up to three months.

Cauliflower Dip

Mix in high-powered blender:

1 head steamed or roasted cauliflower
2 Tbsp ground sesame seeds
2 Tbsp ground sunflower seeds
2 Tbsp olive oil
1 garlic clove
Juice from 1 lemon
Dash of sea salt and black pepper
⅛ tsp each of cumin, paprika, turmeric

Chicken and Veggie Stir Fry

Combine in large fry pan or wok:

½ C cooked lentils or other legume
1 C spinach
2 C sautéed veggies of your choosing (e.g., broccoli, green beans, asparagus, fennel, okra)
2 oz sautéed chicken
2 Tbsp cashew cheese sauce* for topping

Chicken Salad (may substitute salmon or other fish for chicken)

2 oz chicken, cooked
½ C each of cucumber, onion, and tomato
⅓ C adzuki beans, cooked (or whole grain rice, quinoa, lentils)
2 tsp each cilantro, mint, basil, finely chopped
2 C spinach and other vegetables, raw, chopped or shredded (e.g. carrots, cabbage, beets, etc.)
¼ C nuts, seeds, chopped
1 avocado, chopped (alternatively, mash and add to ingredients to hold ingredients together)
1 tsp tarragon, basil, ginger, dill (or your favorites)
Salt to taste
Optional topping: 1 Tbsp nut/seed sauce*

Mix ingredients in a bowl. Top with nut/seed sauce, chopped parsley, or chopped cilantro if desired.

Chicken and Wild Rice Soup

4 C vegetable* or chicken broth*
2 C vegetables, chopped (e.g., carrots, broccoli, rutabaga, fennel, cabbage, cauliflower, beets, turnips, radishes)
1 C leafy greens, chopped (parsley, kale, chard, cilantro, basil, spinach, dandelion greens, arugula)
1 red onion, chopped
2 stalks celery, chopped
1 C chopped chicken
2 cloves garlic, chopped
½ C wild rice
1 Tbsp avocado oil
¼ tsp of each: ground fresh ginger, cumin, fenugreek seed (or sage, thyme, oregano, rosemary, turmeric, etc.)

Put a large saucepan on medium heat on the stove. When hot, add avocado oil, onions and celery. Stir and add herbs and spices. Sauté for 5 minutes until soft. Add chicken and brown slightly. Add broth and bring to boil. Add rice and simmer for 30 minutes. Add vegetables and cook for additional 10–15 minutes. Add leafy greens to serving bowl, ladle hot soup into bowl and serve.

Cookie

1 C of combination of nuts and seeds
1 egg
1 Tbsp pumpkin or squash
1 tsp cinnamon
1 Tbsp coconut oil (unrefined)

Preheat oven to 300°F. Add ingredients to high-powered blender and blend until mixed. Spoon onto greased cookie sheet. Bake at 300°F for 15–20 minutes or until brown.

Crepes (see Waffle)

Date Syrup

3 dates
1 slice beet
1 kale leaf, or spinach, dandelion green
Pinch of cinnamon, clove, nutmeg, cardamon
Water

Add ingredients to high-powered blender. Add water to desired texture for syrup. Use on top of waffles, muffins, crepes, porridge, granola, trail mix.

Flatbread

1 C combination of ground grain, seeds, or nuts (e.g., ⅓ C buckwheat
   groats, ⅓ C flaxseeds, and ⅓ C of pecans ground using a grinder)
¼ tsp baking soda
1 Tbsp juice from lemon
⅔ C water
¼ tsp Himalayan or sea salt
Optional ingredients: oregano, rosemary, thyme, black pepper, sage,
   chopped garlic, ground mustard seed, ground cumin

Preheat oven to 300°F. Add ground flour, baking soda, salt, herbs to
bowl and mix. Combine water and lemon in a measuring cup. Slowly
add liquid to dry ingredients, adjusting the amounts until the mixture
is a dough that you can roll into a ball. Place dough ball between two
pieces of parchment paper. Place on a baking sheet and roll to desired
thickness. Remove the top paper and bake in oven for 25 minutes or
until toasted. Add desired toppings.

Granola (see Trail Mix)

Hearty Bite Muffins

4 large eggs
2 dates
⅓ C organic coconut oil (melted)
1 C organic raw, hulled pumpkin seeds
1 C organic sunflower seeds
3 C organic steamed or baked squash, pumpkin, or sweet potato
1 tsp baking soda (Bob's Red Mill is a good option)
¾ tsp ground organic cinnamon
½ tsp ground organic nutmeg
¼ tsp ground organic ginger
⅛ tsp ground cloves
¼ tsp sea salt

Preheat oven to 350°F. In a high-powered blender, blend wet ingredients and pumpkin seeds. Mix dry ingredients and slowly add to wet ingredient mixture. Blend until smooth. Pour batter into lined mini-muffin tins. Bake until firm, about 50 minutes.

Homemade Flour

Combine 2 C of whole grains, seeds, and nuts (e.g., buckwheat groats, flaxseeds, pecans). Grind ingredients using a coffee grinder or Vitamix dry container. Sift if a finer texture is desired. Adjust ingredients to make up desired volume of flour.

Ice Cream

1 C frozen fruit
½ C seed or nut combo
Water enough to blend
⅛ tsp cinnamon

Add ingredients to high-powered blender and blend until smooth. Put in freezer for 30 minutes, stirring occasionally, until desired consistency.

Kale Quinoa Salad

1 C quinoa, cooked and cooled
1 bunch of kale, stems removed and chopped
1 C roasted vegetables, chopped (e.g., beets, squash, yams, sweet
    potato, rutabaga, turnips, cauliflower, fennel, celery root)
2 C raw vegetables, finely chopped or shredded (broccoli, carrots,
    parsley, cilantro, basil, spinach, chard, arugula, cabbage)
1 lemon, squeezed
1 Tbsp extra-virgin olive oil
Salt to taste

In large salad bowl, add chopped kale, salt, lemon juice, and olive oil. With hands, massage kale until tender. Add assortment of vegetables and mix. Top with nut/seed sauce or tahini dressing.

Marinara Sauce

1 onion, chunked
3 cloves garlic
2 medium carrots, chunked
1 small beet
1 bunch of kale
4 basil leaves
2 tsp each oregano, rosemary, thyme
Salt and black pepper to taste
4 tomatoes (or diced tomatoes in carton)
1 Tbsp extra-virgin olive oil

Add ingredients to high-powered blender and blend on high until smooth. Place sauce in saucepan and simmer for 20–30 minutes. Salt and pepper to taste.

Nut/Seed Butters

2 C combination of nuts and seeds (e.g., pecans, walnuts, Brazil nuts, almonds, hazelnuts, sunflower seeds, pumpkin seeds, flaxseeds)
2 Tbsp avocado oil (or coconut oil)
Salt to taste

Toast nuts on a baking sheet for 5 minutes at 300° F. Then add layer of seeds and toast for another 3–5 minutes. Add toasted nuts and seeds, oil, and salt to high-powered blender. Start low and work up to high and blend to desired texture. Add more oil if blend is dry.

Nut Cheese/Seed Sauces and Spreads (I use this as a cheese replacement)

1 C various seeds and nuts, lightly toasted
1 clove garlic
salt to taste
Optional: add herbs for various tastes (cumin, cayenne, ginger, thyme, rosemary, oregano, fenugreek seed, mustard seed, dill, tarragon, basil, etc.). For example, my Thai spice sauce contains

1 Tbsp whole coriander seeds, 2 tsp whole cumin seeds, 1 tsp whole cardamom seeds, ½ tsp whole cloves, ½ tsp whole black peppercorns, ¼ tsp ground nutmeg, 1 tsp turmeric, 1 tsp dried crushed red pepper

Add water to desired texture (note: thicker blends can be spread on crackers and a thinner version used as a sauce or dressing). Add carrot or a chunk of orange beet for a more "cheesy" orange color. Blend ingredients in high-powered blender for 1 minute.

Nut, Seed, or Grain Milks

1 C any variety of nut, seed, grain, unsweetened coconut dried flakes, or fresh coconut (shredded)
2 C water
Cinnamon (optional)

Blend on high 1 minute in high-powered blender. Strain through cheese or nut cloth or bag. It is okay to use unstrained coconut milk in cooking, for example, when preparing a coconut curry sauce.

Pizza

Make flatbread according to the recipe. Top with homemade marinara sauce* and nut/seed sauce*. Bake at 300°F for 5 minutes. You can top with baked chicken, fresh basil, roasted broccoli, or other vegetables.

Porridge

1 C combined whole grains (e.g., buckwheat groats, oat groats or steel-cut oats, quinoa, millet seeds)
⅓ C chopped fruit/berries
⅓ C nuts or seeds, ground or chopped (e.g., walnut, pecans, pumpkin seeds, sunflower seeds)
Optional ingredients: cinnamon, nutmeg, allspice, cloves, ground vanilla, ginger, turmeric, or other favorites

Rinse grains well and add to 2 C boiling water in saucepan. Turn heat to simmer and let cook until grains are tender, approximately 15–20 minutes. Take off heat and mix in seeds, nuts, fruits, and herbs. If desired, top with date syrup.*

Protein Bar

1 C variety of nuts and seeds
1 date
1 Tbsp coconut oil
Optional: 1 Tbsp cacao or 1 square dark chocolate, 2 oz coconut
   flakes, 2 oz currants

Preheat oven to 350°F. Blend ingredients in high-powered blender. You can add an egg to make blending easier. Mix in optional ingredients by hand. Roll into 1-inch balls and flatten into squares using a fork. Bake for 15 minutes or until toasted.

Savory Flax/Seed Crackers

1 C ground flaxseed (or use a mixture of seeds, e.g., sesame, sunflower,
   pumpkin, flax, chia, hemp)
2 Tbsp onion, finely chopped
1 clove garlic, finely chopped
1 tsp rosemary, ground
1 tsp thyme, ground
½ tsp salt
½ C water
(If you want crackers for nut butters, leave out herbs and add
   cinnamon, nutmeg, cloves, and/or cardamom)

Mix dry ingredients and then add enough water to make a dough ball (you will need to adjust the amount of water according to the seeds used). Place the dough ball between two pieces of parchment paper on sheet and roll out to no more than ¼-inch thick. Remove top paper sheet and cut or score square crackers. Bake at 300°F for about 25 minutes or until toasted on top. Time varies depending on thickness of cracker.

Smoothie Basics

2 C vegetables
½ C fruits
3 herbs (parsley, basil, cilantro, cinnamon, ginger, turmeric, cloves, nutmeg)
¼ C of nuts and seeds (try 1 Tbsp each of two nuts and two seeds)
Water to desired texture
Ice to desired temperature

Blend with high-powered blender.

Smoothie: Veggie-licious

2 C spinach, kale, watercress, dandelion greens, beet greens
1 stalk fennel
¼ C cilantro or parsley
1 tsp each ginger and turmeric
1 Tbsp flaxseeds
1 Tbsp pecans (or walnuts, almonds, hazelnuts)
¼ lemon wedge with rind
½ C fresh or frozen fruit
Water to desired texture
Ice to desired temperature

Blend with high-powered blender.

Smoothie: Berry Fusion

½ C frozen berries
½ cucumber
¼ wedge of beet

1 C leafy greens (e.g., kale, spinach, arugula, dandelion greens, beet greens, parsley, cilantro)
¼ C cabbage
1 celery stalk
1 Tbsp flaxseeds
1 Tbsp sunflower seeds
1 Tbsp almonds
¼ inch ginger slice
⅛ tsp cinnamon
⅛ lemon wedge with rind
Water to desired texture
Ice to desired temperature

Blend with high-powered blender.

Squash Cocoa and Cinnamon Date Nibble

Butternut squash (baked)
½ tsp cocoa powder
1 date
½ tsp cinnamon
⅛ tsp cloves
1 Tbsp coconut oil
salt to taste

Preheat oven to 350°F. To prepare baked squash, cube and bake until tender. Alternatively, cut squash in half and place cut-side down on baking sheet, saving seeds and pulp for smoothie. Bake until tender. Blend oil, spices, and date in a blender, and top squash with mixture.

Tahini Dressing

1 C toasted sesame seeds (toast raw seed in toaster oven for 5 minutes at 300 °F)
Alternatives: sunflower seed, flax, hemp, pumpkin, nuts

3 Tbsp avocado oil or olive oil
1 pinch salt
Optional herbs: mustard seeds, basil, parsley, rosemary, garlic, oregano, fenugreek, cayenne

Blend until smooth.

Tahini, Lemon Juice, and Nut Cheese Dressing

2 cloves garlic
2 Tbsp homemade tahini dressing*
2 Tbsp nut cheese sauce*
2 Tbsp juice from lemon
⅓ C extra virgin olive oil
½ tsp sea salt
3 Tbsp fresh parsley
2 Tbsp water

Put ingredients in high-powered blender and blend until smooth.

Tahini and Mustard Dressing

To Tahini Dressing, add 1 tsp of mustard seed, ground. Optional: add 1 date for more of a sweet-mustard sauce. Put ingredients in high-powered blender and blend until smooth.

Tortilla

½ C ground flaxseeds (I use a coffee grinder dedicated to grinding seeds, nuts, herbs, and grains)
½ C ground buckwheat groats
⅓ C unsweetened coconut flakes
¼ tsp baking soda
squeeze of lemon
⅔ C water
¼ tsp Himalayan or sea salt

Mix in bowl or add ingredients to blender and blend for 1 minute on high. Drop ¼ inch rounds onto a heated, oiled skillet and flatten with a spatula. (Tortillas can also be rolled out before putting in pan.) Fry on medium heat using avocado oil. Cook 2–3 minutes on each side. Adjust heat if browning too quickly on edges.

Trail Mix or Grain-Free Granola

2 C nuts, chopped (almonds, hazelnuts, pecans, etc.)
2 C unsweetened coconut flakes
½ C ground flaxseed (or pumpkin, sunflower, hemp, etc.)
¼ C chopped dates or currants
2 Tbsp coconut oil (raw, unrefined)
1 tsp vanilla extract
½ tsp of ground cinnamon
Optional: ground cloves, grated ginger, cardamom, nutmeg, cayenne
     pepper)

Combine all the ingredients in a bowl and mix. An option is to top the mixture with sliced apple or pear before placing in oven. Place mixture on a baking sheet lined with parchment paper and bake at 350°F for about 25 minutes.

Vegetable Curry Bowl

Curry Sauce:
2 Tbsp olive oil
1 onion, chunked
2 cloves garlic
1 Tbsp fresh ginger
1 tsp cumin seeds
1 tsp coriander seeds
1 tsp turmeric
1 tsp garam masala
½ tsp chili powder
½ tsp salt

3 tomatoes
1 C coconut flakes
2 C vegetables, chopped
2 Tbsp chopped fresh cilantro for topping
½ C cooked brown or wild rice

In a blender, add ingredients for curry sauce and blend on high until smooth. Pour curry sauce into a skillet and simmer on low heat for 10 minutes. Add 2 C chopped vegetables and simmer for about 10 minutes until cooked. Serve over rice and top with fresh chopped cilantro.

Vegetable Fritter

½ C buckwheat groats, ground (I grind the groats first to make flour using a coffee grinder, but you can also add unground groats directly to the blender to make the batter)
1 Tbsp sesame seed, ground
1 Tbsp flaxseed, ground
½ C raw sweet potato, grated
¼ C raw golden beet, shredded (or carrot, parsnips, rutabaga, cabbage)
2 eggs
¼ tsp each of cinnamon and cloves (or for savory, add oregano, rosemary, thyme, sage, and garlic)
salt to taste
Optional: add 1 oz shredded cooked meat or lentils for variety

Add dry ingredients and mix. Add in remainder of ingredients, mix, and make into patties. You can add more ground buckwheat groats if too wet. Pan-fry or bake at 350°F until cooked through.

Waffles/Crepes

2 C homemade flour* from nuts or seeds
3 eggs
¼ C wheat grass (or other green)
¼ C beets (or other vegetable)

½ tsp turmeric
½ tsp cinnamon
¼ tsp cardamom
¼ tsp ground vanilla
salt to taste (pinch)
approximately 1 C water or homemade almond milk (adjust liquid to
    reach desired batter texture)

Blend all ingredients in Vitamix or suitable blender to make batter.
Pour into waffle iron. To make crepes, add more water and pour a thin
layer into a preheated, oiled skillet, flipping when browned on one side.
Optional: for sweeter waffles, add 2 dates; for savory crepes, add savory
spices like rosemary, thyme, and oregano.

Note that with a Vitamix blender, you can make batters from scratch
using whole ingredients. For example, for waffle batter, I'll combine
whole seeds, nuts, and grains in my Vitamix to make a flavorful base.
A base might consist of ½ C flaxseeds, ½ C buckwheat groats, ¼ C
oat groats, and ¼ C pecans. If you don't have a Vitamix, you can grind
whole ingredients in a coffee grinder to make flour and then add to an
ordinary blender with the rest of the ingredients.

Although the food ideas described here only briefly outline what a
full-on REID lifestyle entails, I hope it will inspire you to bring more
whole foods, variety, and all-important vegetables into your diet.
Internet sources are great ways to learn how to prepare unfamiliar
foods, and the knowledge you have gained by reading this book will
suggest ways to make healthy substitutions for inflammatory ingredients included in many online recipes. For example, instead of a mayon-
naise-based dip for roasted artichokes, you might choose a cauliflower
dip. Again, the overarching principles that should guide your selections
are to avoid processed foods, avoid foods enriched with glutamate or
its analogs, avoid or limit wheat and dairy, embrace whole foods, and
celebrate variety.

Are you ready to go shopping? Check out Table B.2 and don't forget
the veggies!

Table B.2. Eat Your Veggies (A through Z)

A	J	S
artichoke, asparagus, arugula, acorn squash	jicama, Jerusalem artichoke	squash, spinach, shallots, sweet potatoes
B beets, broccoli, broccoli rabe, broccolini, brussels sprouts, bok choy, butternut squash, bell peppers	**K** kohlrabi, kale	**T** turnips, taro root
C cabbage, cauliflower, celery, carrot, collard greens, celery root	**L** leeks, lettuces, lima beans, lotus root	**U** ullucus, upland cress
D daikon, dandelion leaves	**M** mustard greens, mushrooms	**V** vigna beans, violets
E eggplant, endive, escarole	**N** nopales, nettles	**W** watercress, watermelon radish, wheatgrass, wasabi
F fava beans, fennel, French beans, fiddleheads	**O** okra, onions	**X** xaxim, xocati squash
G green beans, garlic, gourd	**P** parsnips, potatoes, parsley, pumpkin	**Y** yams, yucca root
H horseradish, hubbard squash	**Q** quelites	**Z** zinnia, zucchini
I Italian parsley	**R** radishes, romanesco, rutabaga, radicchio	

ACKNOWLEDGMENTS

THIS WAS NOT AN EASY BOOK TO WRITE, AND WE ARE GRATEFUL TO everyone who provided encouragement and inspiration. We thank them for the talks about food and health, the exhaustive scientific discussions, and even the sometimes mind-blowing conversations about poop and the trillions of microbial inhabitants residing within our guts. We especially thank the families and friends who have their own special needs kids or health issues and who, by sharing their stories, convinced us this was a book we had to write.

We thank the readers of the early drafts, who gave us critical feedback that helped improve the book. We thank those who conveyed their enthusiasm for the project and their ideas about how to get published. Although not a complete list, we acknowledge the following individuals: Jennifer Balboni, John Bond, Gayle Brubaker Bridges, Lisa Chirnitch, Jeanne Clothiaux, Stacy Frank, Meena Garg, Kanica Gera, Brad Handzel, Maria Mead, Cathy Murphy, Tammy Pelstring, Marc Randolph, Charles Reid, Monica Tomlinson, Andi Stowe, and Hannah Vail.

We thank scientific illustrator Jay McElroy for his simple and elegant drawings.

I, Katherine Reid, am greatly appreciative of my family, who have supported me by believing in my mission and (often unwittingly) serving as recipe testers. A special, loving thank you to:

My youngest daughter, "Taylor," for providing the impetus of my food awakening and nudging my ever-increasing consciousness.

My eldest children, Caitlynn and Reid, for their participation in the journey—through thick and thin.

My sister, Margo, for joining the deep dive food and science conversations while she fights her own health battle.

My mother, Elizabeth, for pressuring me to get this book out before she passed.

And to Barbara Price, my partner in writing this book: I very much enjoyed our many conversations that flowed from thoughts and ideas to words on the page. We did it!

I, Barbara Price, owe a special debt of gratitude to my husband, John McCombs, who believed in this book from the beginning and continues to be its steadfast champion. I thank my sister, Cathy Moore, MS, RD, CDN, for her unflagging support and insight into the nutritional challenges that exist in poor rural communities. And a special shout-out to the incomparable Wendy Rae Johnson, friend and influencer, for her advocacy. Thank you.

From both of us, to all who touched the contents of this book, a heartfelt thank you for your company along the journey. Be well!

NOTES

Introduction

1. Jill Bolte Taylor, *My Stroke of Insight: A Brain Scientist* (New York: Viking, 2006); Norman Doidge, *The Brain That Changes Itself: Stories of Personal Triumph from the Frontiers of Brain Science* (Melbourne: Scribe, 2007).

2. Mark Hyman, *The UltraMind Solution: Fix Your Broken Brain by Healing Your Body First: The Simple Way to Defeat Depression, Overcome Anxiety, and Sharpen Your Mind* (New York: Scribner, 2009).

Chapter 1

1. Recent evidence links glutamate and dopamine as pleasure rewards, and both are linked to addiction wiring in brains. Silas A. Buck et al., "Roles of Dopamine and Glutamate Co-Release in the Nucleus Accumbens in Mediating the Actions of Drugs of Abuse," *FEBS Journal* 288, no. 5 (August 11, 2020): 1462–74, doi:10.1111/febs.15496.

2. Maia Research Co., Ltd., "Global Monosodium Glutamate Production and Consumption from 2021–2022." 2022.

3. Centers for Disease Control and Prevention, "FastStats: Overweight Prevalence," 2019, https://www.cdc.gov/nchs/fastats/obesity-overweight.htm.

4. Centers for Disease Control and Prevention, "FastStats"; Centers for Disease Control and Prevention, "National Diabetes Statistics Report, 2017 Estimates of Diabetes and Its Burden in the United States Background," 2020, https://www.cdc.gov/diabetes/pdfs/data/statistics/national-diabetes-statistics -report.pdf.

5. Centers for Disease Control and Prevention, "Health Policy Data Requests—Percent of U.S. Adults 55 and Over with Chronic Conditions," 2020, https://www.cdc.gov/nchs/health_policy/adult_chronic_conditions.htm.

6. Johns Hopkins Medicine, "Mental Health Disorder Statistics," 2019, https://www.hopkinsmedicine.org/health/wellness-and-prevention/mental -health-disorder-statistics.

7. As reported by parents, during the study period 2009–2017. These included autism, attention deficit/hyperactivity disorder, blindness, and cerebral palsy, among others. Centers for Disease Control and Prevention, "Data & Statistics on Autism Spectrum Disorder," December 2, 2021, https://www.cdc.gov/ncbddd/autism/data.html.

8. Substance Abuse and Mental Health Services Administration, "Results from the 2020 National Survey on Drug Use and Health: Detailed Tables," table 5.1A, Department of Health and Human Services, 2020, https://www.samhsa.gov/data/report/2020-nsduh-detailed-tables.

9. Xiaojia Chen et al., "Consumption of Ultra-Processed Foods and Health Outcomes: A Systematic Review of Epidemiological Studies," *Nutrition Journal* 19, no. 1 (August 20, 2020), doi:10.1186/s12937-020-00604-1; Eduardo A. F. Nilson et al., "Premature Deaths Attributable to the Consumption of Ultraprocessed Foods in Brazil," *American Journal of Preventive Medicine* 64, no. 1 (January 2023): 129–36, doi:10.1016/j.amepre.2022.08.013.

10. Marialaura Bonaccio et al., "Joint Association of Food Nutritional Profile by Nutri-Score Front-of-Pack Label and Ultra-Processed Food Intake with Mortality: Moli-Sani Prospective Cohort Study," *BMJ* 378 (August 31, 2022): e070688, doi:10.1136/bmj-2022-070688; Lu Wang et al., "Association of Ultra-Processed Food Consumption with Colorectal Cancer Risk among Men and Women: Results from Three Prospective US Cohort Studies," *BMJ* 378 (August 31, 2022): e068921, doi:10.1136/bmj-2021-068921.

11. Anaïs Rico-Campà et al., "Association between Consumption of Ultra-Processed Foods and All Cause Mortality: SUN Prospective Cohort Study," *BMJ* 365 (May 29, 2019): l1949, doi:10.1136/bmj.l1949.

Chapter 2

1. M. Afifi and Amr Abbas, "Monosodium Glutamate versus Diet Induced Obesity in Pregnant Rats and Their Offspring," *Acta Physiologica Hungarica* 98, no. 2 (June 2011): 177–88, doi:10.1556/aphysiol.98.2011.2.9; A. E. Hirata et al., "Monosodium Glutamate (MSG)–Obese Rats Develop Glucose Intolerance and Insulin Resistance to Peripheral Glucose Uptake," *Brazilian Journal of Medical and Biological Research* 30, no. 5 (May 1997): 671–667, doi:10.1590/s0100-879x1997000500016.

2. Chiaki Sano, "History of Glutamate Production," *American Journal of Clinical Nutrition* 90, no. 3 (July 29, 2009): 728S732S, doi:10.3945/ajcn.2009.27462f.

3. Jordan Sand, "A Short History of MSG: Good Science, Bad Science, and Taste Cultures," *Gastronomica* 5, no. 4 (November 2005): 38–49, doi:10.1525/gfc.2005.5.4.38.

4. Ichiro Shibuya and Tetsuji Odani, "Method for Producing Amino-Acid-Rich Yeast," Google Patents, November 8, 2008, https://www.google.com/patents/EP2348100A1.

5. Michael Moss, "The Extraordinary Science of Addictive Junk Food," *New York Times Magazine*, February 20, 2013, https://www.nytimes.com/2013/02/24/magazine/the-extraordinary-science-of-junk-food.html.

6. U.S. Food and Drug Administration, "Questions and Answers on Monosodium Glutamate (MSG)," February 20, 2020, http://www.fda.gov/Food/IngredientsPackagingLabeling/FoodAdditivesIngredients/ucm328728.htm.

7. U.S. Food and Drug Administration, "21CFR Part101 Food Labeling," 2008, https://www.govinfo.gov/content/pkg/CFR-2008-title21-vol2/xml/CFR-2008-title21-vol2-part101.xml.

8. TruthHurts315, "MSG on 60 Minutes (1991)," YouTube video, February 11, 2011, https://www.youtube.com/watch?v=8bwBfpWT1PU.

9. Jesus A. Fernandez-Tresguerres Hernández, "Effect of Monosodium Glutamate Given Orally on Appetite Control (a New Theory for the Obesity Epidemic)," *Anales de La Real Academia Nacional de Medicina* 122, no. 2 (2005): 341–55 (discussion 355–360), http://www.ncbi.nlm.nih.gov/pubmed/16463577; Geoffrey R. Skurray and Nicholas Pucar, "L-Glutamic Acid Content of Fresh and Processed Foods," *Food Chemistry* 27, no. 3 (January 1988): 177–80, doi:10.1016/0308-8146(88)90060-x ; T. Populin et al., "A Survey on the Presence of Free Glutamic Acid in Foodstuffs, with and without Added Monosodium Glutamate," *Food Chemistry* 104, no. 4 (2007): 1712–17, doi:10.1016/j.foodchem.2007.03.034.

10. Yoshitaka Toyomasu et al., "Intragastric Monosodium L-Glutamate Stimulates Motility of Upper Gut via Vagus Nerve in Conscious Dogs," *American Journal of Physiology-Regulatory, Integrative and Comparative Physiology* 298, no. 4 (April 2010): R1125–35, doi:10.1152/ajpregu.00691.2009.

11. Food and Drug Administration, "Questions and Answers on Monosodium Glutamate (MSG)."

12. International Food Information Council, "Everything You Need to Know about Glutamate and Monosodium Glutamate," Food Insight, October 17, 2009, https://foodinsight.org/everything-you-need-to-know-about-glutamate-and-monosodium-glutamate.

13. M. Khairunnisak et al., "Monitoring of Free Glutamic Acid in Malaysian Processed Foods, Dishes and Condiments," *Food Additives & Contaminants: Part A* 26, no. 4 (April 2009): 419–26, doi:10.1080/02652030802596860.

14. John W. Olney, "Excitotoxic Food Additives: Functional Teratological Aspects," *Progress in Brain Research*, 1988, 283–94, doi:10.1016/s0079-6123(08) 60510-5.

15. John W. Olney and Oi-Lan Ho, "Brain Damage in Infant Mice Following Oral Intake of Glutamate, Aspartate or Cysteine," *Nature* 227, no. 5258 (August 1970): 609–11, doi:10.1038/227609b0.

16. Akira Niijima, "Reflex Effects of Oral, Gastrointestinal and Hepatoportal Glutamate Sensors on Vagal Nerve Activity," *Journal of Nutrition* 130, no. 4 (April 1, 2000): 971S973S, doi:10.1093/jn/130.4.971s; L. A. Blackshaw et al., "Sensory Transmission in the Gastrointestinal Tract," *Neurogastroenterology & Motility* 19, no. s1 (January 2007): 1–19, doi:10.1111/j.1365-2982.2006.00871.x.

Chapter 3

1. D. R. Lucas and J. P. Newhouse, "The Toxic Effect of Sodium L-Glutamate on the Inner Layers of the Retina," *Archives of Ophthalmology* 58, no. 2 (August 1, 1957): 193–201, doi:10.1001/archopht.1957.00940010205006.

2. J. W. Olney, "Brain Lesions, Obesity, and Other Disturbances in Mice Treated with Monosodium Glutamate," *Science (New York, N.Y.)* 164, no. 3880 (1969): 719–21, doi:10.1126/science.164.3880.719.

3. J. W. Olney, N. J. Adamo, and A. Ratner, "Monosodium Glutamate Effects," *Science* 172, no. 3980 (April 16, 1971): 294–94, doi:10.1126/science .172.3980.294; John W. Olney et al., "Acute Glutamate-Induced Elevations in Serum Testosterone and Luteinizing Hormone," *Brain Research* 112, no. 2 (August 1976): 420–24, doi:10.1016/0006-8993(76)90298-5; John W. Olney, Chandra H. Misra, and Vesa Rhee, "Brain and Retinal Damage from Lathyrus Excitotoxin, β-N-Oxalyl-L-α,β-Diaminopropionic Acid," *Nature* 264, no. 5587 (December 1976): 659–61, doi:10.1038/264659a0; J. W. Olney and L. G. Sharpe, "Brain Lesions in an Infant Rhesus Monkey Treated with Monosodium Glutamate," *Science* 166, no. 3903 (October 17, 1969): 386–88, doi:10.1126 /science.166.3903.386; John W. Olney, Oi Lan Ho, and Vesela Rhee, "Brain-Damaging Potential of Protein Hydrolysates," *New England Journal of Medicine* 289, no. 8 (August 23, 1973): 391–95, doi:10.1056/nejm197308232890802; John W. Olney, "Excitatory Amino Acids and Neuropsychiatric Disorders," *Biological Psychiatry* 26, no. 5 (September 1989): 505–25, doi:10.1016/0006 -3223(89)90072-3; J. W. Olney, "Excitotoxin-Mediated Neuron Death in Youth and Old Age," *Progress in Brain Research* 86 (1990): 37–51, doi:10.1016 /s0079-6123(08)63165-9.

4. Thomas G. Neltner et al., "Navigating the U.S. Food Additive Regulatory Program," *Comprehensive Reviews in Food Science and Food Safety* 10, no. 6

(October 25, 2011): 342–68, doi:10.1111/j.1541-4337.2011.00166.x; Thomas G. Neltner et al., "Conflicts of Interest in Approvals of Additives to Food Determined to Be Generally Recognized as Safe," *JAMA Internal Medicine* 173, no. 22 (December 9, 2013): 2032, doi:10.1001/jamainternmed.2013.10559.

5. Marion Nestle, "Conflicts of Interest in the Regulation of Food Safety," *JAMA Internal Medicine* 173, no. 22 (December 9, 2013): 2036, doi:10.1001 /jamainternmed.2013.9158.

6. Tonkla Insawang et al., "Monosodium Glutamate (MSG) Intake Is Associated with the Prevalence of Metabolic Syndrome in a Rural Thai Population," *Nutrition & Metabolism* 9, no. 1 (2012): 50, doi:10.1186/1743 -7075-9-50; Ka He et al., "Consumption of Monosodium Glutamate in Relation to Incidence of Overweight in Chinese Adults: China Health and Nutrition Survey (CHNS)," *American Journal of Clinical Nutrition* 93, no. 6 (April 6, 2011): 1328–36. doi:10.3945/ajcn.110.008870; M. Hermanussen et al., "Obesity, Voracity, and Short Stature: The Impact of Glutamate on the Regulation of Appetite," *European Journal of Clinical Nutrition* 60, no. 1 (August 31, 2005): 25–31, doi:10.1038/sj.ejcn.1602263.

7. Michael D. Rogers, "Further Studies Are Necessary in Order to Conclude a Causal Association between the Consumption of Monosodium L-Glutamate (MSG) and the Prevalence of Metabolic Syndrome in the Rural Thai Population," *Nutrition & Metabolism* 10, no. 1 (2013): 14, doi:10.1186/1743 -7075-10-14; R. G. Bursey, L. Watson, and M. Smriga, "A Lack of Epidemiologic Evidence to Link Consumption of Monosodium L-Glutamate and Obesity in China," *American Journal of Clinical Nutrition* 94, no. 3 (August 19, 2011): 958– 60, doi:10.3945/ajcn.111.020727.

8. Alison K. Ventura, Gary K. Beauchamp, and Julie A Mennella, "Infant Regulation of Intake: The Effect of Free Glutamate Content in Infant Formulas," *American Journal of Clinical Nutrition* 95, no. 4 (February 22, 2012): 875–81, doi:10.3945/ajcn.111.024919.

9. L. D. Stegink, G. L. Baker, and L. J. Filer, "Modulating Effect of Sustagen on Plasma Glutamate Concentration in Humans Ingesting Monosodium L-Glutamate," *American Journal of Clinical Nutrition* 37, no. 2 (February 1, 1983): 194–200, doi:10.1093/ajcn/37.2.194.

10. Guo-Du Wang et al., "Dietary Glutamate: Interactions with the Enteric Nervous System," *Journal of Neurogastroenterology and Motility* 20, no. 1 (January 31, 2014): 41–53, doi:10.5056/jnm.2014.20.1.41.

11. Bursey et al., "A Lack of Epidemiologic Evidence to Link Consumption of Monosodium L-Glutamate and Obesity in China."

12. C. A. Gobatto et al., "The Monosodium Glutamate (MSG) Obese Rat as a Model for the Study of Exercise in Obesity," *Research Communications in Molecular*

Pathology and Pharmacology 111, no. 1–4 (2002): 89–101, http://www.ncbi.nlm.nih.gov/pubmed/14632317; M. S. Islam and D. T. Loots, "Experimental Rodent Models of Type 2 Diabetes: A Review," *Methods and Findings in Experimental and Clinical Pharmacology* 31, no. 4 (2009): 249, doi:10.1358/mf.2009.31.4.1362513; Koichi Tsuneyama et al., "Neonatal Monosodium Glutamate Treatment Causes Obesity, Diabetes, and Macrovesicular Steatohepatitis with Liver Nodules in DIAR Mice," *Journal of Gastroenterology and Hepatology* 29, no. 9 (August 25, 2014): 1736–43, doi:10.1111/jgh.12610.

13. Kevin D. Hall et al., "Ultra-Processed Diets Cause Excess Calorie Intake and Weight Gain: An Inpatient Randomized Controlled Trial of Ad Libitum Food Intake," *Cell Metabolism* 30, no. 1 (July 2019): 226, doi:10.1016/j.cmet.2019.05.020. For an easy-to-read account of this study, see Ellen Ruppel Shell, "A New Theory of Obesity," *Scientific American*, October 2019, doi:10.1038/scientificamerican1019-38.

14. J. Lexchin, "Pharmaceutical Industry Sponsorship and Research Outcome and Quality: Systematic Review," *BMJ* 326, no. 7400 (May 29, 2003): 1167–70, doi:10.1136/bmj.326.7400.1167; M. Friedberg et al., "Evaluation of Conflict of Interest in Economic Analyses of New Drugs Used in Oncology," *JAMA* 282, no. 15 (October 20, 1999): 1453–57, doi:10.1001/jama.282.15.1453.

15. Naomi Oreskes and Erik M. Conway, *Merchants of Doubt: How a Handful of Scientists Obscured the Truth on Issues from Tobacco Smoke to Global Warming* (New York: Bloomsbury Publishing USA, 2010).

16. Jerry D. Smith et al., "Relief of Fibromyalgia Symptoms Following Discontinuation of Dietary Excitotoxins," *Annals of Pharmacotherapy* 35, no. 6 (June 2001): 702–6, doi:10.1345/aph.10254; Alfred L. Scopp, "MSG and Hydrolyzed Vegetable Protein Induced Headache: Review and Case Studies," *Headache: The Journal of Head and Face Pain* 31, no. 2 (February 1991): 107–10, doi:10.1111/j.1526-4610.1991.hed3102107.x; Yuko Nakanishi et al., "Monosodium Glutamate (MSG): A Villain and Promoter of Liver Inflammation and Dysplasia," *Journal of Autoimmunity* 30, no. 1 (February 1, 2008): 42–50, doi:10.1016/j.jaut.2007.11.016.

17. Some of these authors include George R. Schwartz, who wrote *In Bad Taste: The MSG Symptom Complex: How Monosodium Glutamate Is a Major Cause of Treatable and Preventable Illnesses, such as Headaches, Asthma, Epilepsy, Heart Irregularities, Depression, Rage Reactions, and Attention Deficit Hyperactivity Disorder* (Santa Fe, NM: Health Press, 1999), and Russell L. Blaylock, *Excitotoxins: The Taste That Kills* (Santa Fe, NM: Health Press, 1998). Russel Blaylock is a retired neurosurgeon medical doctor with a stated mission in his book to raise awareness of the health issues associated with MSG in food. Adrienne Samuels, PhD, a psychologist, has been raising awareness on MSG in food for multiple

decades. She established the Truth in Labeling organization and has written letters to the FDA and journals regarding some gross errors and lack of transparency in glutamate industry-funded clinical trials on MSG safety. Her publications include *The Perfect Poison* (Adrienne Samuels, 2022), *The Man Who Sued the FDA* (Adrienne Samuels, 2013), and "The Toxicity/Safety of Processed Free Glutamic Acid (MSG): A Study in Suppression of Information," *Accountability in Research* 6, no. 4 (July 1999): 259–310, doi:10.1080/08989629908573933. Carol Hoernlein is the founder of MSGtruth.org established to raise awareness to consumers. See also John E. Erb and T. Michelle Erb, *The Slow Poisoning of America* (Virginia Beach, Va.: Paladins Press, 2003).

18. FDA Letters, "You Have the Right to Know What Is in Your Food," Citizens Petition # 94P-0444, Food and Drug Administration, Department of Health and Human Services, September 15, 1995; John Erb, "Revoke the GRAS Standing of the Food Additive Monosodium Glutamate," Citizens Petition FDA-2007-P-0178-0002, Food and Drug and Administration, Department of Health and Human Services, 2008; Michael Landa, "FDA/CFSAN to John Erb—Petition Denial, FDA-2007-P-0178," Food and Drug Administration. Department of Health and Human Services, 2012.

Chapter 4

1. See Susannah Cahalan, *Brain on Fire* (New York: Simon and Schuster, 2013). Susannah makes a connection between her type of encephalitis (an autoimmune disease) and glutamate dysregulation. In her case, the targets of the disease-causing agent (antibodies) were glutamate receptors in the brain.

2. Md Abdul Alim et al., "Glutamate Triggers the Expression of Functional Ionotropic and Metabotropic Glutamate Receptors in Mast Cells," *Cellular & Molecular Immunology* 18, no. 10 (April 20, 2020): 2383–92, doi:10.1038 /s41423-020-0421-z.

3. Niamh M. C. Connolly and Jochen H. M. Prehn, "The Metabolic Response to Excitotoxicity—Lessons from Single-Cell Imaging," *Journal of Bioenergetics and Biomembranes* 47, no. 1–2 (September 28, 2014): 75–88, doi:10.1007/s10863-014-9578-4.

4. John W. Olney, "Excitotoxic Food Additives: Functional Teratological Aspects," *Progress in Brain Research*, 1988, 283–94, doi:10.1016/s0079-6123 (08)60510-5.

5. J. W. Olney, "Excitotoxic Food Additives—Relevance of Animal Studies to Human Safety," *Neurobehavioral Toxicology and Teratology* 6, no. 6 (November 1, 1984): 455–62, http://www.ncbi.nlm.nih.gov/pubmed/6152304.

6. Yann Bernardinelli, Irina Nikonenko, and Dominique Muller, "Structural Plasticity: Mechanisms and Contribution to Developmental Psychiatric Disorders," *Frontiers in Neuroanatomy* 8 (November 3, 2014): 123, doi:10.3389/fnana.2014.00123.

7. Victor A. Derkach et al., "Regulatory Mechanisms of AMPA Receptors in Synaptic Plasticity," *Nature Reviews Neuroscience* 8, no. 2 (February 2007): 101–13, doi:10.1038/nrn2055.

8. John Prescott, "Effects of Added Glutamate on Liking for Novel Food Flavors," *Appetite* 42, no. 2 (April 2004): 143–50, doi:10.1016/j.appet.2003.08.013.

9. France Bellisle, "Glutamate and the UMAMI Taste: Sensory, Metabolic, Nutritional and Behavioural Considerations. A Review of the Literature Published in the Last 10 Years," *Neuroscience & Biobehavioral Reviews* 23, no. 3 (January 1, 1999): 423–38, doi:10.1016/S0149-7634(98)00043-8.

10. Julie A. Mennella et al., "Early Milk Feeding Influences Taste Acceptance and Liking during Infancy," *American Journal of Clinical Nutrition* 90, no. 3 (July 15, 2009): 780S788S, doi:10.3945/ajcn.2009.27462o.

11. Kunio Torii, Hisayuki Uneyama, and Eiji Nakamura, "Physiological Roles of Dietary Glutamate Signaling via Gut–Brain Axis Due to Efficient Digestion and Absorption," *Journal of Gastroenterology* 48, no. 4 (March 6, 2013): 442–51, doi:10.1007/s00535-013-0778-1.

Chapter 5

1. See, for example, Ed Yong, *I Contain Multitudes: The Microbes within Us and a Grander View of Life* (New York: Ecco, 2018).

2. Lu Gao et al., "Oral Microbiomes: More and More Importance in Oral Cavity and Whole Body," *Protein & Cell* 9, no. 5 (May 2018): 488–500, doi:10.1007/s13238-018-0548-1.

3. John Prescott, "Effects of Added Glutamate on Liking for Novel Food Flavors," *Appetite* 42, no. 2 (April 2004): 143–50, doi:10.1016/j.appet.2003.08.013.

4. Nobuhiro Takahashi, Takuichi Sato, and Tadashi Yamada, "Metabolic Pathways for Cytotoxic End Product Formation from Glutamate- and Aspartate-Containing Peptides by *Porphyromonas Gingivalis*," *Journal of Bacteriology* 182, no. 17 (September 2000): 4704–10, doi:10.1128/jb.182.17.4704-4710.2000.

5. Saher S. Mohammed, "Monosodium Glutamate-Induced Genotoxicity in Rat Palatal Mucosa," *Tanta Dental Journal* 14, no. 3 (2017): 112, doi:10.4103/tdj.tdj_20_17.

6. Peter J. Turnbaugh et al., "The Human Microbiome Project," *Nature* 449, no. 7164 (October 18, 2007): 804–10, doi:10.1038/nature06244.

7. Moises Velasquez-Manoff, *An Epidemic of Absence: A New Way of Understanding Allergies and Autoimmune Diseases* (New York: Scribner, 2013).

8. Andrew C. Dukowicz, Brian E. Lacy, and Gary M. Levine, "Small Intestinal Bacterial Overgrowth: A Comprehensive Review," *Gastroenterology & Hepatology* 3, no. 2 (February 1, 2007): 112–22, https://www.ncbi.nlm.nih.gov /pubmed/21960820.

9. K. Aagaard et al., "The Placenta Harbors a Unique Microbiome," *Science Translational Medicine* 6, no. 237 (May 21, 2014): 237ra65–65, doi:10.1126 /scitranslmed.3008599.

10. C. De Filippo et al., "Impact of Diet in Shaping Gut Microbiota Revealed by a Comparative Study in Children from Europe and Rural Africa," *Proceedings of the National Academy of Sciences* 107, no. 33 (August 2, 2010): 14691–96, doi:10.1073/pnas.1005963107.

11. Turnbaugh et al., "The Human Microbiome Project."

12. Peter J. Turnbaugh et al., "A Core Gut Microbiome in Obese and Lean Twins," *Nature* 457, no. 7228 (November 30, 2008): 480–84, doi:10.1038 /nature07540.

13. Christopher L. Gentile and Tiffany L. Weir, "The Gut Microbiota at the Intersection of Diet and Human Health," *Science* 362, no. 6416 (November 15, 2018): 776–80, doi:10.1126/science.aau5812; Michael Conlon and Anthony Bird, "The Impact of Diet and Lifestyle on Gut Microbiota and Human Health," *Nutrients* 7, no. 1 (December 24, 2014): 17–44, doi:10.3390 /nu7010017; Lawrence A. David et al., "Diet Rapidly and Reproducibly Alters the Human Gut Microbiome," *Nature* 505, no. 7484 (December 11, 2013): 559–63, doi:10.1038/nature12820; Ian Rowland et al., "Gut Microbiota Functions: Metabolism of Nutrients and Other Food Components," *European Journal of Nutrition* 57, no. 1 (April 9, 2017): 1–24, doi:10.1007/s00394-017-1445-8.

14. R. H. Yolken and E. F. Torrey, "Are Some Cases of Psychosis Caused by Microbial Agents? A Review of the Evidence," *Molecular Psychiatry* 13, no. 5 (May 1, 2008): 470–79, doi:10.1038/mp.2008.5; Michael Karin, Toby Lawrence, and Victor Nizet, "Innate Immunity Gone Awry: Linking Microbial Infections to Chronic Inflammation and Cancer," *Cell* 124, no. 4 (February 2006): 823–35, doi:10.1016/j.cell.2006.02.016; R. J. Xavier, and D. K. Podolsky, "Unravelling the Pathogenesis of Inflammatory Bowel Disease," *Nature* 448, no. 7152 (July 2007): 427–34, doi:10.1038/nature06005; J. F. Cryan and S. M. O'Mahony, "The Microbiome–Gut–Brain Axis: From Bowel to Behavior," *Neurogastroenterology & Motility* 23, no. 3 (February 8, 2011): 187–92, doi:10.1111/j.1365-2982.2010.01664.x.

15. F. Backhed, "Host-Bacterial Mutualism in the Human Intestine," *Science* 307, no. 5717 (March 25, 2005): 1915–20, doi:10.1126/science.1104816.

16. Ze-Meng Feng et al., "Monosodium L-Glutamate and Dietary Fat Differently Modify the Composition of the Intestinal Microbiota in Growing Pigs," *Obesity Facts* 8, no. 2 (2015): 87–100, doi:10.1159/000380889.

17. L. V. Hooper, "Molecular Analysis of Commensal Host-Microbial Relationships in the Intestine," *Science* 291, no. 5505 (February 2, 2001): 881–84, doi:10.1126/science.291.5505.881; Ruixin Liu et al., "Gut Microbiome and Serum Metabolome Alterations in Obesity and after Weight-Loss Intervention," *Nature Medicine* 23, no. 7 (June 19, 2017): 859–68, doi:10.1038/nm.4358.

18. Filip Ottosson et al., "Connection between BMI-Related Plasma Metabolite Profile and Gut Microbiota," *Journal of Clinical Endocrinology & Metabolism* 103, no. 4 (February 1, 2018): 1491–1501, doi:10.1210/jc.2017-02114.

19. Feng et al., "Monosodium L-Glutamate and Dietary Fat Differently Modify the Composition of the Intestinal Microbiota in Growing Pigs"; Oleksandr A. Savcheniuk et al., "The Efficacy of Probiotics for Monosodium Glutamate-Induced Obesity: Dietology Concerns and Opportunities for Prevention," *EPMA Journal* 5, no. 1 (January 13, 2014), doi:10.1186/1878-5085-5-2.

20. J. J. Faith et al., "Predicting a Human Gut Microbiota's Response to Diet in Gnotobiotic Mice," *Science* 333, no. 6038 (May 19, 2011): 101–4, doi:10.1126/science.1206025.

21. R. Hughes, E. A. Magee, and S. Bingham, "Protein Degradation in the Large Intestine: Relevance to Colorectal Cancer," *Current Issues in Intestinal Microbiology* 1, no. 2 (September 1, 2000): 51–58, http://www.ncbi.nlm.nih.gov/pubmed/11709869.

22. Elaine Holmes et al., "Understanding the Role of Gut Microbiome–Host Metabolic Signal Disruption in Health and Disease," *Trends in Microbiology* 19, no. 7 (July 2011): 349–59, doi:10.1016/j.tim.2011.05.006; A. Ruhl, "Glial Cells in the Gut," *Neurogastroenterology and Motility* 17, no. 6 (December 2005): 777–90, doi:10.1111/j.1365-2982.2005.00687.x; Keith A. Sharkey and Alfons B.A. Kroese, "Consequences of Intestinal Inflammation on the Enteric Nervous System: Neuronal Activation Induced by Inflammatory Mediators," *Anatomical Record* 262, no. 1 (January 1, 2001): 79–90, doi:10.1002/1097-0185(20010101)262:1<79::aid-ar1013>3.0.co;2-k; Emeran A. Mayer, Kirsten Tillisch, and Arpana Gupta, "Gut/Brain Axis and the Microbiota," *Journal of Clinical Investigation* 125, no. 3 (February 17, 2015): 926–38, doi:10.1172/jci76304.

23. T. D. Prickett and Y. Samuels, "Molecular Pathways: Dysregulated Glutamatergic Signaling Pathways in Cancer," *Clinical Cancer Research* 18, no. 16 (May 30, 2012): 4240–46, doi:10.1158/1078-0432.ccr-11-1217. There is a

nutrient consequence, too, as detoxification requires sulfation, leaving the host depleted of sulfur, which is necessary to protect cells.

24. Jennifer S. Labus et al., "Evidence for an Association of Gut Microbial Clostridia with Brain Functional Connectivity and Gastrointestinal Sensorimotor Function in Patients with Irritable Bowel Syndrome, Based on Tripartite Network Analysis," *Microbiome* 7, no. 1 (March 21, 2019), doi:10.1186/s40168-019-0656-z.

25. Andreina Baj et al., "Glutamatergic Signaling along the Microbiota-Gut-Brain Axis," *International Journal of Molecular Sciences* 20, no. 6 (March 25, 2019): 1482, doi:10.3390/ijms20061482.

26. Mitsuharu Matsumoto et al., "Cerebral Low-Molecular Metabolites Influenced by Intestinal Microbiota: A Pilot Study," *Frontiers in Systems Neuroscience* 7 (2013), doi:10.3389/fnsys.2013.00009; Takahiro Kawase et al., "Gut Microbiota of Mice Putatively Modifies Amino Acid Metabolism in the Host Brain," *British Journal of Nutrition* 117, no. 6 (March 1, 2017): 775–83, doi:10.1017/S0007114517000678.

27. Arpana Gupta, Vadim Osadchiy, and Emeran A. Mayer, "Brain–Gut–Microbiome Interactions in Obesity and Food Addiction," *Nature Reviews Gastroenterology & Hepatology* 17, no. 11 (August 27, 2020): 655–72, doi:10.1038/s41575-020-0341-5.

28. Cryan and O'Mahony, "The Microbiome–Gut–Brain Axis"; Ruth Ann Luna and Jane A Foster, "Gut Brain Axis: Diet Microbiota Interactions and Implications for Modulation of Anxiety and Depression," *Current Opinion in Biotechnology* 32 (April 2015): 35–41, doi:10.1016/j.copbio.2014.10.007; Gerard Sanacora, Giulia Treccani, and Maurizio Popoli, "Towards a Glutamate Hypothesis of Depression," *Neuropharmacology* 62, no. 1 (January 2012): 63–77, doi:10.1016/j.neuropharm.2011.07.036; Dennis J. McCarthy et al., "Glutamate-Based Depression GBD," *Medical Hypotheses* 78, no. 5 (May 2012): 675–81, doi:10.1016/j.mehy.2012.02.009.

29. Marisa Iati, "He Was Acting Drunk but Swore He Was Sober. Turns out His Stomach Was Brewing Its Own Beer," *Washington Post*, October 30, 2019, https://www.washingtonpost.com/health/2019/10/24/he-was-acting-drunk-swore-he-was-sober-turns-out-his-stomach-was-brewing-its-own-beer/.

Chapter 6

1. A. K. Walker et al., "Neuroinflammation and Comorbidity of Pain and Depression," *Pharmacological Reviews* 66, no. 1 (December 11, 2013): 80–101, doi:10.1124/pr.113.008144.

2. Hakan Alfredson and Ronny Lorentzon, "Chronic Tendon Pain: No Signs of Chemical Inflammation but High Concentrations of the Neurotransmitter Glutamate. Implications for Treatment?" *Current Drug Targets* 3, no. 1 (February 1, 2002), doi:10.2174/1389450023348028.

3. Ebrahim Haroon, Andrew H. Miller, and Gerard Sanacora, "Inflammation, Glutamate, and Glia: A Trio of Trouble in Mood Disorders," *Neuropsychopharmacology* 42, no. 1 (September 15, 2016): 193–215, doi:10.1038/npp.2016.199.

4. Hind Abdo et al., "Specialized Cutaneous Schwann Cells Initiate Pain Sensation," *Science* 365, no. 6454 (August 15, 2019): 695–99, doi:10.1126/science.aax6452.

5. Kathleen F. Holton, Peter K. Ndege, and Daniel J. Clauw, "Dietary Correlates of Chronic Widespread Pain in Meru, Kenya," *Nutrition* 53 (September 2018): 14–19, doi:10.1016/j.nut.2018.01.016.

6. Holton et al., "Dietary Correlates of Chronic Widespread Pain"; Julie Wieseler-Frank, Steven F Maier, and Linda R Watkins, "Glial Activation and Pathological Pain," *Neurochemistry International* 45, no. 2–3 (2004): 389–95, doi:10.1016/j.neuint.2003.09.009.

7. Zumin Shi et al., "Monosodium Glutamate Is Related to a Higher Increase in Blood Pressure over 5 Years: Findings from the Jiangsu Nutrition Study of Chinese Adults," *Journal of Hypertension* 29, no. 5 (May 2011): 846–53, doi:10.1097/hjh.0b013e328344da8e; Laura J. Stevens et al., "Dietary Sensitivities and ADHD Symptoms: Thirty-Five Years of Research," *Clinical Pediatrics* 50, no. 4 (December 2, 2010): 279–93, doi:10.1177/0009922810384728; Jean-Claude Moubarac et al., "Consumption of Ultra-Processed Foods and Likely Impact on Human Health: Evidence from Canada," *Public Health Nutrition* 16, no. 12 (November 21, 2012): 2240–48, doi:10.1017/s1368980012005009; Kathleen Feeney Holton et al., "Novel Dietary Intervention Produces Significant Improvements in Fibromyalgia Patients with Irritable Bowel Syndrome," *FASEB Journal* 24, no. S1 (April 2010), doi:10.1096/fasebj.24.1_supplement.564.23; Makoto Fujimoto et al., "A Dietary Restriction Influences the Progression but Not the Initiation of MSG-Induced Nonalcoholic Steatohepatitis," *Journal of Medicinal Food* 17, no. 3 (March 2014): 374–83, doi:10.1089/jmf.2012.0029; Kate S. Collison et al., "Effect of Dietary Monosodium Glutamate on HFCS-Induced Hepatic Steatosis: Expression Profiles in the Liver and Visceral Fat," *Obesity* 18, no. 6 (June 2010): 1122–34, doi:10.1038/oby.2009.502; Jerry D. Smith et al., "Relief of Fibromyalgia Symptoms Following Discontinuation of Dietary Excitotoxins," *Annals of Pharmacotherapy* 35, no. 6 (June 2001): 702–6, doi:10.1345/aph.10254; Robert Dantzer and Adam K. Walker, "Is There a Role for Glutamate-Mediated Excitotoxicity in Inflammation-Induced Depression?"

Journal of Neural Transmission 121, no. 8 (March 15, 2014): 925–32, doi:10.1007/s00702-014-1187-1.

8. Some of these studies were in mice, showing that MSG directly contributed to a particular source of inflammation even when other items in the diet were controlled. Other studies showed MSG contributed to inflammatory conditions in humans, and still other studies showed that the elimination of MSG helped manage particular inflammatory conditions. One of the goals of the Unblind My Mind nonprofit I started is to secure enough funding to do a double-blind study examining the effectiveness of REID in an autism population.

9. Researchers are studying glutamate-based depression—not so much for the purpose of making dietary recommendations but to develop drugs that block glutamate binding to cell receptors. I recommend trying food options first.

10. Ellen A. Lumpkin and Michael J. Caterina, "Mechanisms of Sensory Transduction in the Skin," *Nature* 445, no. 7130 (February 2007): 858–65, doi:10.1038/nature05662; Timothy M. Skerry and Paul G. Genever, "Glutamate Signalling in Non-Neuronal Tissues," *Trends in Pharmacological Sciences* 22, no. 4 (April 2001): 174–81, doi:10.1016/s0165-6147(00)01642-4.

11. Justin Sonnenburg and Erica Sonnenburg, *The Good Gut* (Random House, 2015).

12. Vladimir Grubišić, et al., "Enteric Glia Regulate Gut Motility in Health and Disease," *Brain Research Bulletin* 136 (January 2018): 109–17, doi:10.1016/j.brainresbull.2017.03.011.

13. Anne Ruhl, "Glial Cells in the Gut," *Neurogastroenterology and Motility* 17, no. 6 (December 2005): 777–90, doi:10.1111/j.1365-2982.2005.00687.x.

14. Julie Cabarrocas, Tor C. Savidge, and Roland S. Liblau, "Role of Enteric Glial Cells in Inflammatory Bowel Disease," *Glia* 41, no. 1 (December 3, 2002): 81–93, doi:10.1002/glia.10169.

15. Min-Tsai Liu et al., "Glutamatergic Enteric Neurons," *Journal of Neuroscience* 17, no. 12 (June 15, 1997): 4764–84, doi:10.1523/jneurosci.17-12-04764.1997; Julie Wieseler-Frank, Steven F Maier, and Linda R. Watkins, "Glial Activation and Pathological Pain," *Neurochemistry International* 45, no. 2–3 (2004): 389–95, doi:10.1016/j.neuint.2003.09.009.

16. Annette L. Kirchgessner, Min-Tsai Liu, and Frederick Alcantara, "Excitotoxicity in the Enteric Nervous System," *Journal of Neuroscience* 17, no. 22 (November 15, 1997): 8804–16, doi:10.1523/jneurosci.17-22-08804.1997.

17. Tor C. Savidge, Michael V. Sofroniew, and Michel Neunlist, "Starring Roles for Astroglia in Barrier Pathologies of Gut and Brain," *Laboratory Investigation* 87, no. 8 (July 2, 2007): 731–36, doi:10.1038/labinvest.3700600; Gabrio Bassotti et al., "Enteric Glial Cells: New Players in Gastrointestinal Motility?" *Laboratory Investigation* 87, no. 7 (May 7, 2007): 628–32, doi:10.1038/labinvest.3700564.

18. Anne Cornet et al., "Enterocolitis Induced by Autoimmune Targeting of Enteric Glial Cells: A Possible Mechanism in Crohn's Disease?" *Proceedings of the National Academy of Sciences of the United States of America* 98, no. 23 (November 6, 2001): 13306–11, doi:10.1073/pnas.231474098; A-C. Aube, "Changes in Enteric Neurone Phenotype and Intestinal Functions in a Transgenic Mouse Model of Enteric Glia Disruption," *Gut* 55, no. 5 (May 1, 2006): 630–37, doi:10.1136/gut.2005.067595.

19. Viviana Filpa et al., "Role of Glutamatergic Neurotransmission in the Enteric Nervous System and Brain-Gut Axis in Health and Disease," *Neuropharmacology* 111 (December 2016): 14–33, doi:10.1016/j.neuropharm.2016.08.024.

20. Holton et al., "Novel Dietary Intervention Produces Significant Improvements in Fibromyalgia Patients."

21. Vasiliy Zolotarev et al., "Effect of Free Dietary Glutamate on Gastric Secretion in Dogs." *Annals of the New York Academy of Sciences* 1170, no. 1 (July 2009): 87–90. doi:10.1111/j.1749-6632.2009.03900.x.

22. Zemeng Feng et al., "Monosodium L-Glutamate and Dietary Fat Exert Opposite Effects on the Proximal and Distal Intestinal Health in Growing Pigs," *Applied Physiology, Nutrition, and Metabolism* 40, no. 4 (April 2015): 353–63, doi:10.1139/apnm-2014-0434.

23. Hans Christian Helms et al., "In Vitro Evidence for the Brain Glutamate Efflux Hypothesis: Brain Endothelial Cells Cocultured with Astrocytes Display a Polarized Brain-To-Blood Transport of Glutamate," *Glia* 60, no. 6 (March 5, 2012): 882–93, doi:10.1002/glia.22321.

24. Even though the molecule glutamate is controlled at the BBB, glutamate signaling is not. In other words, chronic inflammation anywhere in the body sends signals to the brain that can cause the brain to get overexcited and awash in glutamate released from its own neurons. For example, cytokines generated from an inflamed gut will cross the BBB and excite brain cells.

25. N. Joan Abbott, Lars Rönnbäck, and Elisabeth Hansson, "Astrocyte–Endothelial Interactions at the Blood–Brain Barrier," *Nature Reviews Neuroscience* 7, no. 1 (January 2006): 41–53, doi:10.1038/nrn1824; Oliver I. Schmidt et al., "Tumor Necrosis Factor-Mediated Inhibition of Interleukin-18 in the Brain: A Clinical and Experimental Study in Head-Injured Patients and in a Murine Model of Closed Head Injury," *Journal of Neuroinflammation* 1, no. 1 (2004): 13, doi:10.1186/1742-2094-1-13.

26. E. A. van Vliet et al., "Blood-Brain Barrier Leakage May Lead to Progression of Temporal Lobe Epilepsy," *Brain* 130, no. 2 (February 1, 2007): 521–34, doi:10.1093/brain/awl318; V. Rigau et al., "Angiogenesis Is Associated with Blood-Brain Barrier Permeability in Temporal Lobe Epilepsy," *Brain* 130, no. 7 (May 29, 2007): 1942–56, doi:10.1093/brain/awm118; S. Ivens et al., "TGF-beta Receptor-Mediated Albumin Uptake into Astrocytes Is Involved

in Neocortical Epileptogenesis," *Brain* 130, no. 2 (February 1, 2007): 535–47, doi:10.1093/brain/awl317.

27. Sarah L. Smith and Edward D. Hall, "Mild Pre- and Posttraumatic Hypothermia Attenuates Blood-Brain Barrier Damage Following Controlled Cortical Impact Injury in the Rat," *Journal of Neurotrauma* 13, no. 1 (January 1996): 1–9, doi:10.1089/neu.1996.13.1; Huang Upadhyay and R. J. Tamargo, "Inflammation in Stroke and Focal Cerebral Ischemia," *Surgical Neurology* 66, no. 3 (September 1, 2006): 232–45, doi:10.1016/j.surneu.2005.12.028.

28. Angela MacIntyre et al., "*Chlamydia Pneumoniae* Infection Alters the Junctional Complex Proteins of Human Brain Microvascular Endothelial Cells," *FEMS Microbiology Letters* 217, no. 2 (December 2002): 167–72. doi:10.1111/j.1574-6968.2002.tb11470.x; Itai Weissberg et al., "Blood-Brain Barrier Dysfunction in Epileptogenesis of the Temporal Lobe," *Epilepsy Research and Treatment* 2011 (June 7, 2011): 1–10, doi:10.1155/2011/143908.

29. Interestingly, in the first year of life, the blood-brain barrier of infants is relatively permeable. All the more reason to limit the fortification of baby formula with excitotoxins like glutamate!

30. Marcela Julio-Pieper et al., "Exciting Times beyond the Brain: Metabotropic Glutamate Receptors in Peripheral and Non-Neural Tissues," *Pharmacological Reviews* 63, no. 1 (January 12, 2011): 35–58, doi:10.1124/pr.110.004036.

31. Jessica L. F. Teh and Suzie Chen, "Glutamatergic Signaling in Cellular Transformation," *Pigment Cell & Melanoma Research* 25, no. 3 (February 20, 2012): 331–42. doi:10.1111/j.1755-148x.2012.00983.x.

32. Shu-Heng Jiang et al., "Neurotransmitters: Emerging Targets in Cancer," *Oncogene* 39, no. 3 (September 16, 2019): 503–15, doi:10.1038/s41388-019-1006-0.

33. Richard G. Bakker et al., "Identification of Specific Chemoattractants and Genetic Complementation of a *Borrelia burgdorferi* Chemotaxis Mutant: Flow Cytometry-Based Capillary Tube Chemotaxis Assay," *Applied and Environmental Microbiology* 73, no. 4 (February 15, 2007): 1180–88, doi:10.1128/aem.01913-06.

34. Sébastien Bontemps-Gallo, Kevin Lawrence, and Frank C. Gherardini, "Two Different Virulence-Related Regulatory Pathways in Borrelia Burgdorferi Are Directly Affected by Osmotic Fluxes in the Blood Meal of Feeding Ixodes Ticks," *PLoS Pathogens* 12, no. 8 (August 15, 2016): e1005791, doi:10.1371/journal.ppat.1005791.

35. Anna M. Hansen and Rachel R Caspi, "Glutamate Joins the Ranks of Immunomodulators," *Nature Medicine* 16, no. 8 (August 2010): 856–58, doi:10.1038/nm0810-856.

Chapter 7

1. Zach Snitzer, "40M Americans Met Criteria for Substance Use Disorder in 2020: MARC," Maryland Addiction Recovery Center, November 1, 2021, https://www.marylandaddictionrecovery.com/40-million-americans-substance-use-disorder-2020/.

2. Centers for Disease Control and Prevention, "Drug Overdose Deaths in the U.S. Top 100,000 Annually," November 17, 2021, https://www.cdc.gov/nchs/pressroom/nchs_press_releases/2021/20211117.htm.

3. American Psychiatric Association, *Diagnostic and Statistical Manual of Mental Disorders* (5th ed.) (American Psychiatric Publishing, Inc., 2013), https://doi.org/10.1176/appi.books.9780890425596.

4. Barbara H. Herman, *Glutamate and Addiction* (Springer Science & Business Media, 2002).

5. Joachim D. Uys and Kathryn J. Reissner, "Glutamatergic Neuroplasticity in Cocaine Addiction," *Progress in Molecular Biology and Translational Science* (2011): 367–400, doi:10.1016/b978-0-12-385506-0.00009-0.

6. Wenhan Yang et al., "Increased Absolute Glutamate Concentrations and Glutamate-to-Creatine Ratios in Patients with Methamphetamine Use Disorders," *Frontiers in Psychiatry* 9 (August 31, 2018), doi:10.3389/fpsyt.2018.00368.

7. National Institute on Alcohol Abuse and Alcoholism, "Alcohol Facts and Statistics," March 2022, https://www.niaaa.nih.gov/publications/brochures-and-fact-sheets/alcohol-facts-and-statistics.

8. P. Kalivas, "Glutamate Systems in Cocaine Addiction," *Current Opinion in Pharmacology* 4, no. 1 (February 2004): 23–29, doi:10.1016/j.coph.2003.11.002; Dana Most, Laura Ferguson, and R. Adron Harris, "Molecular Basis of Alcoholism," *Handbook of Clinical Neurology*, 2014, 89–111. doi:10.1016/b978-0-444-62619-6.00006-9.

9. Amaia M. Erdozain and Luis F. Callado, "Neurobiological Alterations in Alcohol Addiction: A Review," *Adicciones* 26, no. 4 (2014): 360–70, http://www.ncbi.nlm.nih.gov/pubmed/25578004.

10. John Olney, "Fetal Alcohol Syndrome at the Cellular Level," *Addiction Biology* 9, no. 2 (June 2004): 137–49, doi:10.1080/13556210410001717006.

11. Sophie E. Holmes et al., "Altered Metabotropic Glutamate Receptor 5 Markers in PTSD: In Vivo and Postmortem Evidence," *Proceedings of the National Academy of Sciences*, July 12, 2017, doi:10.1073/pnas.1701749114.

12. Bessel van der Kolk et al., "Inescapable Shock, Neurotransmitters, and Addiction to Trauma: Toward a Psychobiology of Post Traumatic Stress," *Biological Psychiatry* 20, no. 3 (March 1985): 314–25, doi:https://doi.org/10.1016/0006-3223(85)90061-7.

13. Centers for Disease Control and Prevention, "Alzheimer's Disease and Related Dementias," October 26, 2020, https://www.cdc.gov/aging/aginginfo/alzheimers.htm.

14. William F. Maragos et al., "Glutamate Dysfunction in Alzheimer's Disease: An Hypothesis," *Trends in Neurosciences* 10, no. 2 (February 1987): 65–68, doi:10.1016/0166-2236(87)90025-7.

15. M. Hynd, "Glutamate-Mediated Excitotoxicity and Neurodegeneration in Alzheimer's Disease," *Neurochemistry International* 45, no. 5 (October 2004): 583–95, doi:10.1016/j.neuint.2004.03.007; Carolyn C. Rudy et al., "The Role of the Tripartite Glutamatergic Synapse in the Pathophysiology of Alzheimer's Disease," *Aging and Disease* 6, no. 2 (2015): 131, doi:10.14336/ad.2014.0423.

16. Hyoung-gon Lee et al., "The Role of Metabotropic Glutamate Receptors in Alzheimer's Disease," *Acta Neurobiologiae Experimentalis* 64, no. 1 (2004): 89–98, http://www.ncbi.nlm.nih.gov/pubmed/15190683.

17. Olakunle James Onaolapo, Olaleye Samuel Aremu, and Adejoke Yetunde Onaolapo, "Monosodium Glutamate-Associated Alterations in Open Field, Anxiety-Related and Conditioned Place Preference Behaviours in Mice," *Naunyn-Schmiedeberg's Archives of Pharmacology* 390, no. 7 (March 29, 2017): 677–89, doi:10.1007/s00210-017-1371-6.

18. Centers for Disease Control and Prevention, "Data and Statistics about ADHD," September 23, 2021. https://www.cdc.gov/ncbddd/adhd/data.html.

19. Gail Tripp and Jeffery R. Wickens, "Neurobiology of ADHD," *Neuropharmacology* 57, no. 7–8 (December 2009): 579–89, doi:10.1016/j.neuropharm.2009.07.026.

20. Jayne Cartmell and Darryle D. Schoepp, "Regulation of Neurotransmitter Release by Metabotropic Glutamate Receptors," *Journal of Neurochemistry* 75, no. 3 (January 4, 2002): 889–907, doi:10.1046/j.1471-4159.2000.0750889.x.

21. Gabriele Ende et al., "Impulsivity and Aggression in Female BPD and ADHD Patients: Association with ACC Glutamate and GABA Concentrations," *Neuropsychopharmacology* 41, no. 2 (June 4, 2015): 410–18, doi:10.1038/npp.2015.153; Jochen Bauer et al., "Hyperactivity and Impulsivity in Adult Attention-Deficit/Hyperactivity Disorder Is Related to Glutamatergic Dysfunction in the Anterior Cingulate Cortex," *World Journal of Biological Psychiatry* 19, no. 7 (December 15, 2016): 538–46, doi:10.1080/15622975.2016.1262060.

22. Jos. J. Eggermont and Larry E. Roberts, "The Neuroscience of Tinnitus: Understanding Abnormal and Normal Auditory Perception," *Frontiers in Systems Neuroscience* 6 (2012), doi:10.3389/fnsys.2012.00053.

23. Raelyn Janssen, Laura Schweitzer, and Karl F. Jensen, "Glutamate Neurotoxicity in the Developing Rat Cochlea: Physiological and Morphological Approaches," *Brain Research* 552, no. 2 (June 1991): 255–64, doi:10.1016/0006-8993(91)90090-i.

24. Lidy M. Pelsser et al., "Effects of a Restricted Elimination Diet on the Behaviour of Children with Attention-Deficit Hyperactivity Disorder (INCA Study): A Randomised Controlled Trial," *The Lancet* 377, no. 9764 (February 2011): 494–503, doi:10.1016/s0140-6736(10)62227-1.

25. Centers for Disease Control and Prevention, "Data & Statistics on Autism Spectrum Disorder," December 2, 2021, https://www.cdc.gov/ncbddd/autism/data.html.

26. R. Blaylock and A. Strunecka, "Immune-Glutamatergic Dysfunction as a Central Mechanism of the Autism Spectrum Disorders," *Current Medicinal Chemistry* 16, no. 2 (January 1, 2009): 157–70, doi:10.2174/0929867097870027 45; J. L. R. Rubenstein and M. M. Merzenich, "Model of Autism: Increased Ratio of Excitation/Inhibition in Key Neural Systems," *Genes, Brain and Behavior* 2, no. 5 (October 16, 2003): 255–67, doi:10.1034/j.1601-183x.2003.00037.x; Mark S. Brown et al., "Increased Glutamate Concentration in the Auditory Cortex of Persons with Autism and First-Degree Relatives: A1H-MRS Study," *Autism Research* 6, no. 1 (November 16, 2012): 1–10, doi:10.1002/aur.1260; Jennifer E. Siegel-Ramsay et al., "Glutamate and Functional Connectivity-Support for the Excitatory-Inhibitory Imbalance Hypothesis in Autism Spectrum Disorders," *Psychiatry Research: Neuroimaging* 313 (2021): 111302; Sofie De Wandel et al., "Altered Glutamate and Glutamine Kinetics in Autism Spectrum Disorder," *Current Developments in Nutrition* 5, no. Supplement_2 (2021): 845; Greg C. Carlson, "Glutamate Receptor Dysfunction and Drug Targets across Models of Autism Spectrum Disorders," *Pharmacology Biochemistry and Behavior* 100, no. 4 (February 2012): 850–54, doi:10.1016/j.pbb.2011.02.003; Paromita Roy Choudhury, Sanjukta Lahiri, and Usha Rajamma, "Glutamate Mediated Signaling in the Pathophysiology of Autism Spectrum Disorders," *Pharmacology Biochemistry and Behavior* 100, no. 4 (February 2012): 841–49, doi:10.1016/j.pbb.2011.06.023; Pinchen Yang and Chen-Lin Chang, "Glutamate-Mediated Signaling and Autism Spectrum Disorders: Emerging Treatment Targets," *Current Pharmaceutical Design* 20, no. 32 (January 10, 2014): 5186–93, Doi:10.2174/13816128196661401101020725.

27. A. El-Ansary, "GABA and Glutamate Imbalance in Autism and Their Reversal as Novel Hypothesis for Effective Treatment Strategy," *Autism and Developmental Disorders* 18, no. 3 (2020): 46–63, doi:https://doi.org/10.17759/autdd.2020180306; Russell G. Port, Lindsay M. Oberman, and Timothy P. L. Roberts, "Revisiting the Excitation/Inhibition Imbalance Hypothesis of ASD through a Clinical Lens," *British Journal of Radiology* 92, no. 1101 (September 2019): 20180944, doi:10.1259/bjr.20180944.

28. A. E. Purcell et al., "Postmortem Brain Abnormalities of the Glutamate Neurotransmitter System in Autism," *Neurology* 57, no. 9 (November 13, 2001): 1618–28, doi:10.1212/wnl.57.9.1618.

29. Victor A. Derkach et al., "Regulatory Mechanisms of AMPA Receptors in Synaptic Plasticity," *Nature Reviews Neuroscience* 8, no. 2 (February 2007): 101–13, doi:10.1038/nrn2055.

30. Kwok-On Lai and Nancy Y. Ip, "Structural Plasticity of Dendritic Spines: The Underlying Mechanisms and Its Dysregulation in Brain Disorders," *Biochimica et Biophysica Acta (BBA)—Molecular Basis of Disease* 1832, no. 12 (December 1, 2013): 2257–63, doi:10.1016/j.bbadis.2013.08.012.

31. M. M. Essa et al., "Excitotoxicity in the Pathogenesis of Autism," *Neurotoxicity Research* 23, no. 4 (October 13, 2012): 393–400, doi:10.1007 /s12640-012-9354-3.

32. R. K. Naviaux, "Metabolic Features of the Cell Danger Response," *Mitochondrion* 16 (May 1, 2014): 7–17, doi:10.1016/j.mito.2013.08.006; Alan M. Smith et al., "A Metabolomics Approach to Screening for Autism Risk in the Children's Autism Metabolome Project," *Autism Research* 13, no. 8 (June 18, 2020): 1270–85, doi:10.1002/aur.2330.

33. Tore Midtvedt, "The Gut: A Triggering Place for Autism—Possibilities and Challenges," *Microbial Ecology in Health & Disease* 23 (August 24, 2012), doi:10.3402/mehd.v23i0.18982; Dae-Wook Kang et al., "Long-Term Benefit of Microbiota Transfer Therapy on Autism Symptoms and Gut Microbiota," *Scientific Reports* 9, no. 1 (April 9, 2019), doi:10.1038/s41598-019-42183-0.

34. Martha R. Herbert and Karen Weintraub, *The Autism Revolution: Whole-Body Strategies for Making Life All It Can Be* (New York: Ballantine Books, 2012).

35. ACS Medical Content and News Staff, "2022 Cancer Facts & Figures: Cancer Death Rate Drops," American Cancer Society, January 12, 2022, https://www.cancer.org/latest-news/facts-and-figures-2022.html.

36. Rebecca L. Siegel, Kimberly D. Miller, and Ahmedin Jemal, "Cancer Statistics, 2019," *CA: A Cancer Journal for Clinicians* 69, no. 1 (January 2019): 7–34, doi:10.3322/caac.21551.

37. T. Takano et al., "Glutamate Release Promotes Growth of Malignant Gliomas," *Nature Medicine* 7, no. 9 (2001): 1010–15. doi:10.1038/nm0901-1010.

38. Jessica L. F. Teh and Suzie Chen, "Glutamatergic Signaling in Cellular Transformation," *Pigment Cell & Melanoma Research* 25, no. 3 (February 20, 2012): 331–42, doi:10.1111/j.1755-148x.2012.00983.x; T. D. Prickett and Y. Samuels, "Molecular Pathways: Dysregulated Glutamatergic Signaling Pathways in Cancer," *Clinical Cancer Research* 18, no. 16 (May 30, 2012): 4240–46, doi:10.1158/1078-0432.ccr-11-1217.

39. Teh and Chen, "Glutamatergic Signaling in Cellular Transformation."

40. E. Haroon, A. H. Miller, and G. Sanacora, "Inflammation, Glutamate, and Glia: A Trio of Trouble in Mood Disorders," *Neuropsychopharmacology: Official Publication of the American College of Neuropsychopharmacology* 42, no. 1

(January 2017): 193–215, doi:10.1038/npp.2016.199; Anna M. Hansen and Rachel R. Caspi, "Glutamate Joins the Ranks of Immunomodulators," *Nature Medicine* 16, no. 8 (August 2010): 856–58, doi:10.1038/nm0810-856.

41. Teh and Chen, "Glutamatergic Signaling in Cellular Transformation"; Prickett and Samuels, "Molecular Pathways: Dysregulated Glutamatergic Signaling Pathways in Cancer"; Siegel-Ramsay et al., "Glutamate and Functional Connectivity."

42. N. Müller and M. J. Schwarz, "The Immune-Mediated Alteration of Serotonin and Glutamate: Towards an Integrated View of Depression," *Molecular Psychiatry* 12, no. 11 (April 24, 2007): 988–1000, doi:10.1038 /sj.mp.4002006; Hideaki Mitani et al., "Correlation between Plasma Levels of Glutamate, Alanine and Serine with Severity of Depression," *Progress in Neuro-Psychopharmacology and Biological Psychiatry* 30, no. 6 (August 2006): 1155–58, doi:10.1016/j.pnpbp.2006.03.036; A. C. Altamura et al., "Plasma and Platelets Glutamate Levels in Major Psychoses," *Schizophrenia Research* 9, no. 2–3 (April 1993): 215, doi:10.1016/0920-9964(93)90461-q; Kenji Hashimoto, Akira Sawa, and Masaomi Iyo, "Increased Levels of Glutamate in Brains from Patients with Mood Disorders," *Biological Psychiatry* 62, no. 11 (December 2007): 1310–16, doi:10.1016/j.biopsych.2007.03.017; Thomas McGrath et al., "Emerging Evidence for the Widespread Role of Glutamatergic Dysfunction in Neuropsychiatric Diseases," *Nutrients* 14, no. 5 (2022): 917, doi:10.3390 /nu14050917.

43. Leah McNally, Zubin Bhagwagar, and Jonas Hannestad, "Inflammation, Glutamate, and Glia in Depression: A Literature Review," *CNS Spectrums* 13, no. 6 (June 1, 2008): 501–10, doi:10.1017/s1092852900016734; Adejoke Yetunde Onaolapo and Olakunle James Onaolapo, "Glutamate and Depression: Reflecting a Deepening Knowledge of the Gut and Brain Effects of a Ubiquitous Molecule." *World Journal of Psychiatry* 11, no. 7 (2021): 297, doi:10.5498/wjp .v11.i7.297; Cecilie Bay-Richter et al., "A Role for Inflammatory Metabolites as Modulators of the Glutamate N-Methyl-d-Aspartate Receptor in Depression and Suicidality," *Brain, Behavior, and Immunity* 43 (January 2015): 110–17, doi:10.1016/j.bbi.2014.07.012.

44. Dennis J. McCarthy et al., "Glutamate-Based Depression GBD," *Medical Hypotheses* 78, no. 5 (May 2012): 675–81, doi:10.1016/j.mehy.2012.02.009.

45. Centers for Disease Control and Prevention, "National DPP Customer Service Center," 2022, https://nationaldppcsc.cdc.gov/s/article/CDC-2022 -National-Diabetes-Statistics-Report.

46. Filip Ottosson et al., "Altered Asparagine and Glutamate Homeostasis Precede Coronary Artery Disease and Type 2 Diabetes," *Journal of Clinical Endocrinology & Metabolism* 103, no. 8 (May 16, 2018): 3060–69, doi:10.1210

/jc.2018-00546; Manami Oya et al., "Amino Acid Taste Receptor Regulates Insulin Secretion in Pancreatic β-Cell Line MIN6 Cells," *Genes to Cells* 16, no. 5 (April 6, 2011): 608–16, doi:10.1111/j.1365-2443.2011.01509.x.

47. Centers for Disease Control and Prevention, "Adult Obesity Facts," February 11, 2021, https://www.cdc.gov/obesity/data/adult.html.

48. Robin B. Kanarek et al., "Juvenile-Onset Obesity and Deficits in Caloric Regulation in MSG-Treated Rats," *Pharmacology Biochemistry and Behavior* 10, no. 5 (May 1979): 717–21, doi:10.1016/0091-3057(79)90324-1; L. Macho et al., "Late Effects of Postnatal Administration of Monosodium Glutamate on Insulin Action in Adult Rats," *Physiological Research* 49 Suppl 1 (2000): S79–85. http://www.ncbi.nlm.nih.gov/pubmed/10984075; Oleksandr A. Savcheniuk et al., "The Efficacy of Probiotics for Monosodium Glutamate-Induced Obesity: Dietology Concerns and Opportunities for Prevention," *EPMA Journal* 5, no. 1 (January 13, 2014), doi:10.1186/1878-5085-5-2.

49. Tonkla Insawang et al., "Monosodium Glutamate (MSG) Intake Is Associated with the Prevalence of Metabolic Syndrome in a Rural Thai Population," *Nutrition & Metabolism* 9, no. 1 (2012): 50, doi:10.1186/1743-7075-9-50; Ka He et al., "Consumption of Monosodium Glutamate in Relation to Incidence of Overweight in Chinese Adults: China Health and Nutrition Survey (CHNS)," *American Journal of Clinical Nutrition* 93, no. 6 (April 6, 2011): 1328–36, doi:10.3945/ajcn.110.008870.

50. M. Hermanussen et al., "Obesity, Voracity, and Short Stature: The Impact of Glutamate on the Regulation of Appetite," *European Journal of Clinical Nutrition* 60, no. 1 (August 31, 2005): 25–31, doi:10.1038/sj.ejcn.1602263.

51. Ana Andres-Hernando et al., "Umami-Induced Obesity and Metabolic Syndrome Is Mediated by Nucleotide Degradation and Uric Acid Generation," *Nature Metabolism* 3, no. 9 (2021): 1189–1201, doi:10.1038/s42255-021-00454-z. David Perlmutter also writes about the links between uric acid levels and inflammation by this same pathway of nucleotide degradation; see Perlmutter, *Drop Acid* (Hachette UK, 2022).

52. Insawang et al., "Monosodium Glutamate (MSG) Intake Is Associated with the Prevalence of Metabolic Syndrome in a Rural Thai Population"; He et al., "Consumption of Monosodium Glutamate in Relation to Incidence of Overweight in Chinese Adults"; Alberto M. Davalli, Carla Perego, and Franco B. Folli, "The Potential Role of Glutamate in the Current Diabetes Epidemic," *Acta Diabetologica* 49, no. 3 (January 5, 2012): 167–83, doi:10.1007/s00592-011-0364-z; Koichi Tsuneyama et al., "Neonatal Monosodium Glutamate Treatment Causes Obesity, Diabetes, and Macrovesicular Steatohepatitis with Liver Nodules in DIAR Mice," *Journal of Gastroenterology and Hepatology* 29, no. 9 (August 25, 2014): 1736–43, doi:10.1111/jgh.12610.

53. R. G. Bursey, L. Watson, and M. Smriga, "A Lack of Epidemiologic Evidence to Link Consumption of Monosodium L-Glutamate and Obesity in China," *American Journal of Clinical Nutrition* 94, no. 3 (August 19, 2011): 958–60, doi:10.3945/ajcn.111.020727.

54. Abril Oliva Ramirez et al., "Prevalence and Burden of Multiple Sclerosis-Related Fatigue: A Systematic Literature Review," *BMC Neurology* 21, no. 1 (December 2021), doi:10.1186/s12883-021-02396-1.

55. Richard Macrez et al., "Mechanisms of Glutamate Toxicity in Multiple Sclerosis: Biomarker and Therapeutic Opportunities," *The Lancet Neurology* 15, no. 10 (September 2016): 1089–1102, doi:10.1016/s1474-4422(16)30165-x.

56. Russell L. Blaylock, *Multiple Sclerosis* (Atlanta, GA: Pritchett & Hull), 1988; David Pitt, Peter Werner, and Cedric S. Raine, "Glutamate Excitotoxicity in a Model of Multiple Sclerosis," *Nature Medicine* 6, no. 1 (January 2000): 67–70, doi:10.1038/71555; G. Rosati, "The Prevalence of Multiple Sclerosis in the World: An Update," *Neurological Sciences* 22, no. 2 (April 1, 2001): 117–39, doi:10.1007/s100720170011; Christopher Bolton and Carolyn Paul, "Glutamate Receptors in Neuroinflammatory Demyelinating Disease," *Mediators of Inflammation* 2006 (2006): 1–12, doi:10.1155/mi/2006/93684.

57. Massimo Filippi et al., "Association between Pathological and MRI Findings in Multiple Sclerosis," *The Lancet Neurology* 11, no. 4 (April 2012): 349–60, doi:10.1016/s1474-4422(12)70003-0; Stefan D. Roosendaal et al., "Grey Matter Volume in a Large Cohort of MS Patients: Relation to MRI Parameters and Disability," *Multiple Sclerosis* 17, no. 9 (September 1, 2011): 1098–1106. doi:10.1177/1352458511404916.

58. L. Hammit, "Glutamate Identified as Predictor of Disease Progression in Multiple Sclerosis," University of California San Francisco, April 29, 2009, https://www.ucsf.edu/news/2009/04/4227/glutamate-identified-predictor -disease-progression-multiple-sclero.

59. Terry Wahls et al., "Dietary Approaches to Treat MS-Related Fatigue: Comparing the Modified Paleolithic (Wahls Elimination) and Low Saturated Fat (Swank) Diets on Perceived Fatigue in Persons with Relapsing-Remitting Multiple Sclerosis: Study Protocol for a Randomized Controlled Trial," *Trials* 19 (June 4, 2018), doi:10.1186/s13063-018-2680-x.

60. Ruth L. O'Gorman Tuura, Christian R. Baumann, and Heide Baumann-Vogel. "Beyond Dopamine: GABA, Glutamate, and the Axial Symptoms of Parkinson's Disease," *Frontiers in Neurology* 9 (September 26, 2018), doi:10.3389/fneur.2018.00806.

61. Dario Cuomo et al., "Metabotropic Glutamate Receptor Subtype 4 Selectively Modulates Both Glutamate and GABA Transmission in the Striatum: Implications for Parkinson's Disease Treatment," *Journal of Neurochemistry*

109, no. 4 (May 2009): 1096–1105, doi:10.1111/j.1471-4159.2009.06036.x; F. Blandini and J. T. Greenamyre, "Prospects of Glutamate Antagonists in the Therapy of Parkinson's Disease," *Fundamental & Clinical Pharmacology* 12, no. 1 (January 2, 1998): 4–12, doi:10.1111/j.1472-8206.1998.tb00918.x; Fabio Blandini and Marie-Therese Armentero, "New Pharmacological Avenues for the Treatment of L-DOPA-Induced Dyskinesias in Parkinson's Disease: Targeting Glutamate and Adenosine Receptors," *Expert Opinion on Investigational Drugs* 21, no. 2 (January 11, 2012): 153–68, doi:10.1517/13543784.2012.651457.

62. Ji Wang et al., "Molecular Mechanisms of Glutamate Toxicity in Parkinson's Disease," *Frontiers in Neuroscience* 14 (November 26, 2020), doi:10.3389/fnins.2020.585584.

63. B. Meldrum, "Amino Acids as Dietary Excitotoxins: A Contribution to Understanding Neurodegenerative Disorders," *Brain Research Reviews* 18, no. 3 (December 1993): 293–314, doi:10.1016/0165-0173(93)90014-q.

64. Matteo Briguglio et al., "Dietary Neurotransmitters: A Narrative Review on Current Knowledge," *Nutrients* 10, no. 5 (May 10, 2018): 591, doi:10.3390/nu10050591.

65. Golam M. Khandaker and Robert Dantzer, "Is There a Role for Immune-to-Brain Communication in Schizophrenia?" *Psychopharmacology* 233, no. 9 (June 4, 2015): 1559–73, doi:10.1007/s00213-015-3975-1.

66. Laura R. Lachance and Kwame McKenzie, "Biomarkers of Gluten Sensitivity in Patients with Non-Affective Psychosis: A Meta-Analysis." *Schizophrenia Research* 152, no. 2–3 (February 2014): 521–27, doi:10.1016/j.schres.2013.12.001.

67. Norbert Müller, "Inflammation and the Glutamate System in Schizophrenia: Implications for Therapeutic Targets and Drug Development," *Expert Opinion on Therapeutic Targets* 12, no. 12 (November 13, 2008): 1497–1507, doi:10.1517/14728220802507852.

68. Yota Uno and Joseph T. Coyle, "Glutamate Hypothesis in Schizophrenia," *Psychiatry and Clinical Neurosciences* 73, no. 5 (March 6, 2019): 204–15, doi:10.1111/pcn.12823.

69. Peter Jeon et al., "Progressive Changes in Glutamate Concentration in Early Stages of Schizophrenia: A Longitudinal 7-Tesla MRS Study," *Schizophrenia Bulletin Open* 2, no. 1 (January 1, 2021), doi:10.1093/schizbullopen/sgaa072.

70. A. Sherwin et al., "Excitatory Amino Acids Are Elevated in Human Epileptic Cerebral Cortex," *Neurology* 38, no. 6 (June 1, 1988): 920–20, doi:10.1212/wnl.38.6.920.

71. Astrid G. Chapman, "Glutamate and Epilepsy," *Journal of Nutrition* 130, no. 4 (April 1, 2000): 1043S1045S, doi:10.1093/jn/130.4.1043s.

72. Andrew Lutas and Gary Yellen, "The Ketogenic Diet: Metabolic Influences on Brain Excitability and Epilepsy," *Trends in Neurosciences* 36, no. 1 (January 2013): 32–40, doi:10.1016/j.tins.2012.11.005.

73. Marcela Julio-Pieper et al., "Exciting Times beyond the Brain: Metabotropic Glutamate Receptors in Peripheral and Non-Neural Tissues," *Pharmacological Reviews* 63, no. 1 (January 12, 2011): 35–58, doi:10.1124 /pr.110.004036.

74. Jerry D. Smith et al., "Relief of Fibromyalgia Symptoms Following Discontinuation of Dietary Excitotoxins," *Annals of Pharmacotherapy* 35, no. 6 (June 2001): 702–6, doi:10.1345/aph.10254; Kathleen Feeney Holton et al., "Novel Dietary Intervention Produces Significant Improvements in Fibromyalgia Patients with Irritable Bowel Syndrome," *FASEB Journal* 24, no. S1 (April 2010), doi:10.1096/fasebj.24.1_supplement.564.23.

75. J. Gordon Millichap and Michelle M. Yee, "The Diet Factor in Pediatric and Adolescent Migraine," *Pediatric Neurology* 28, no. 1 (January 2003): 9–15, doi:10.1016/s0887-8994(02)00466-6; Alan G. Finkel, Juanita Yerry, and J. Douglas Mann, "Dietary Considerations in Migraine Management: Does a Consistent Diet Improve Migraine?" *Current Pain and Headache Reports* 17, no. 11 (September 26, 2013), doi:10.1007/s11916-013-0373-4.

76. M. Longoni and C. Ferrarese, "Inflammation and Excitotoxicity: Role in Migraine Pathogenesis," *Neurological Sciences* 27, no. S2 (May 2006): s107–10, doi:10.1007/s10072-006-0582-2.

Chapter 8

1. Check out this veterinarian raising awareness of glutamate in pet food: DogtorJ., "DogtorJ.com: Food Intolerance in Pets & Their People: Home of the GARD," 2009, https://dogtorj.com.

2. Katherine Reid, "Katie Reid and Smoothies for Health—Get Started Now,"YouTube video, 2013, https://www.youtube.com/watch?v=4OsoDopmy1k.

3. For ingredients in KFC chicken, see Fooducate, "No Product Found," accessed December 8, 2022, https://www.fooducate.com/product/KFC-Chicken -Pot-Pie/8963DD6E-398F-11E3-A74D-1E047F0525AB; for MSG in fast food restaurants, see NaturalNews, "Busted! KFC, Chick-Fil-A, Burger King and Other Fast Food Restaurants Caught Using Huge Quantities of MSG While Calling Their Menu Items Fresh," accessed December 8, 2022, https:// www.naturalnews.com/KFC-Chick-fil-A-Burger-King-Pizza-Hut-MSG -menu-items.html.

Appendix A

1. Jean-Claude Moubarac et al., "Consumption of Ultra-Processed Foods Predicts Diet Quality in Canada," *Appetite* 108 (January 2017): 512–20, doi:10.1016/j.appet.2016.11.006; Milena Nardocci et al., "Consumption of Ultra-Processed Foods and Obesity in Canada," *Canadian Journal of Public Health = Revue Canadienne de Sante Publique* 110, no. 1 (2019): 4–14, doi:10.17269/s41997-018-0130-x; Anaïs Rico-Campà et al., "Association between Consumption of Ultra-Processed Foods and All Cause Mortality: SUN Prospective Cohort Study," *BMJ* 365 (May 29, 2019): l1949, doi:10.1136/bmj .l1949; Carlos Augusto Monteiro et al., "The UN Decade of Nutrition, the NOVA Food Classification and the Trouble with Ultra-Processing," *Public Health Nutrition* 21, no. 1 (March 21, 2017): 5–17, doi:10.1017/s1368980017000234.

2. Monteiro et al., "The UN Decade of Nutrition."

3. Moubarac et al., "Consumption of Ultra-Processed Foods Predicts Diet Quality in Canada."

4. N. Slimani et al., "Contribution of Highly Industrially Processed Foods to the Nutrient Intakes and Patterns of Middle-Aged Populations in the European Prospective Investigation into Cancer and Nutrition Study," *European Journal of Clinical Nutrition* 63, no. 4 (November 1, 2009): S206–25, doi:10.1038 /ejcn.2009.82; Eurídice Martínez Steele et al., "Ultra-Processed Foods and Added Sugars in the US Diet: Evidence from a Nationally Representative Cross-Sectional Study," *BMJ Open* 6, no. 3 (January 2016): e009892, doi:10.1136 /bmjopen-2015-009892; Pan American Health Organization, "Ultra-Processed Food and Drink Products in Latin America: Trends, Impact on Obesity, Policy Implications" (Washington DC: World Health Organization, 2015), https:// iris.paho.org/bitstream/handle/10665.2/7699/9789275118641_eng.pdf; C. A. Monteiro et al., "Ultra-Processed Products Are Becoming Dominant in the Global Food System," *Obesity Reviews* 14 (October 23, 2013): 21–28, doi:10.1111/obr.12107; Gyorgy Scrinis and Carlos Monteiro, "From Ultra-Processed Foods to Ultra-Processed Dietary Patterns," *Nature Food*, September 15, 2022, doi:10.1038/s43016-022-00599-4.

5. Moubarac et al., "Consumption of Ultra-Processed Foods Predicts Diet Quality in Canada."

6. Serena Niro et al., "Evolution of Free Amino Acids during Ripening of Caciocavallo Cheeses Made with Different Milks," *Journal of Dairy Science* 100, no. 12 (December 2017): 9521–31, doi:10.3168/jds.2017-13308.

7. Moubarac et al., "Consumption of Ultra-Processed Foods Predicts Diet Quality in Canada."

8. C. Thiele, M. G. Gänzle, and R. F. Vogel, "Contribution of Sourdough Lactobacilli, Yeast, and Cereal Enzymes to the Generation of Amino Acids in Dough Relevant for Bread Flavor," *Cereal Chemistry Journal* 79, no. 1 (January 2002): 45–51, doi:10.1094/cchem.2002.79.1.45.

9. Stefan Pasiakos et al., "Sources and Amounts of Animal, Dairy, and Plant Protein Intake of US Adults in 2007–2010," *Nutrients* 7, no. 8 (August 21, 2015): 7058–69, doi:10.3390/nu7085322.

BIBLIOGRAPHY

Aagaard, K., J. Ma, K. M. Antony, R. Ganu, J. Petrosino, and J. Versalovic. "The Placenta Harbors a Unique Microbiome." *Science Translational Medicine* 6, no. 237 (May 21, 2014): 237ra65–65. doi:10.1126/scitranslmed.3008599.

Abbott, N. Joan, Lars Rönnbäck, and Elisabeth Hansson. "Astrocyte–Endothelial Interactions at the Blood–Brain Barrier." *Nature Reviews Neuroscience* 7, no. 1 (January 2006): 41–53. doi:10.1038/nrn1824.

Abdo, Hind, Laura Calvo-Enrique, Jose Martinez Lopez, Jianren Song, Ming-Dong Zhang, Dmitry Usoskin, Abdeljabbar El Manira, Igor Adameyko, Jens Hjerling-Leffler, and Patrik Ernfors. "Specialized Cutaneous Schwann Cells Initiate Pain Sensation." *Science* 365, no. 6454 (August 15, 2019): 695–99. doi:10.1126/science.aax6452.

ACS Medical Content and News Staff. "2022 Cancer Facts & Figures: Cancer Death Rate Drops." American Cancer Society, January 12, 2022. https://www.cancer.org/latest-news/facts-and-figures-2022.html.

Afifi, M., and Amr Abbas. "Monosodium Glutamate versus Diet Induced Obesity in Pregnant Rats and Their Offspring." *Acta Physiologica Hungarica* 98, no. 2 (June 2011): 177–88. doi:10.1556/aphysiol.98.2011.2.9.

Alfredson, Hakan, and Ronny Lorentzon. "Chronic Tendon Pain: No Signs of Chemical Inflammation but High Concentrations of the Neurotransmitter Glutamate: Implications for Treatment?" *Current Drug Targets* 3, no. 1 (February 1, 2002). doi:10.2174/1389450023348028.

Alim, Md Abdul, Mirjana Grujic, Paul W. Ackerman, Per Kristiansson, Pernilla Eliasson, Magnus Peterson, and Gunnar Pejler. "Glutamate Triggers the Expression of Functional Ionotropic and Metabotropic Glutamate Receptors in Mast Cells." *Cellular & Molecular Immunology* 18, no. 10 (April 20, 2020): 2383–92. doi:10.1038/s41423-020-0421-z.

Altamura, A. C., M. C. Mauri, A. Ferrara, and G. D'Andrea. "Plasma and Platelets Glutamate Levels in Major Psychoses." *Schizophrenia Research* 9, nos. 2–3 (April 1993): 215. doi:10.1016/0920-9964(93)90461-q.

American Psychiatric Association. *Diagnostic and Statistical Manual of Mental Disorders*. 5th ed. American Psychiatric Publishing, Inc., 2013. https://doi .org/10.1176/appi.books.9780890425596.

Andres-Hernando, Ana, Christina Cicerchi, Masanari Kuwabara, David J. Orlicky, Laura Gabriela Sanchez-Lozada, Takahiko Nakagawa, Richard J. Johnson, and Miguel A. Lanaspa. "Umami-Induced Obesity and Metabolic Syndrome Is Mediated by Nucleotide Degradation and Uric Acid Generation." *Nature Metabolism* 3, no. 9 (September 2021): 1189– 1201. doi:10.1038/s42255-021-00454-z.

Aube, A-C. "Changes in Enteric Neurone Phenotype and Intestinal Functions in a Transgenic Mouse Model of Enteric Glia Disruption." *Gut* 55, no. 5 (May 1, 2006): 630–37. doi:10.1136/gut.2005.067595.

Backhed, F. "Host-Bacterial Mutualism in the Human Intestine." *Science* 307, no. 5717 (March 25, 2005): 1915–20. doi:10.1126/science.1104816.

Baj, Andreina, Elisabetta Moro, Michela Bistoletti, Viviana Orlandi, Francesca Crema, and Cristina Giaroni. "Glutamatergic Signaling along the Microbiota-Gut-Brain Axis." *International Journal of Molecular Sciences* 20, no. 6 (March 25, 2019): 1482. doi:10.3390/ijms20061482.

Bakker, Richard G., Chunhao Li, Michael R. Miller, Cynthia Cunningham, and Nyles W. Charon. "Identification of Specific Chemoattractants and Genetic Complementation of a *Borrelia burgdorferi* Chemotaxis Mutant: Flow Cytometry-Based Capillary Tube Chemotaxis Assay." *Applied and Environmental Microbiology* 73, no. 4 (February 15, 2007): 1180–88. doi:10.1128/aem.01913-06.

Bassotti, Gabrio, Vincenzo Villanacci, Elisabetta Antonelli, Antonio Morelli, and Bruno Salerni. "Enteric Glial Cells: New Players in Gastrointestinal Motility?" *Laboratory Investigation* 87, no. 7 (May 7, 2007): 628–32. doi:10.1038/labinvest.3700564.

Bauer, Jochen, Anne Werner, Waldemar Kohl, Harald Kugel, Anna Shushakova, Anya Pedersen, and Patricia Ohrmann. "Hyperactivity and Impulsivity in Adult Attention-Deficit/Hyperactivity Disorder Is Related to Glutamatergic Dysfunction in the Anterior Cingulate Cortex." *World Journal of Biological Psychiatry* 19, no. 7 (December 15, 2016): 538–46. doi: 10.1080/15622975.2016.1262060.

Bay-Richter, Cecilie, Klas R. Linderholm, Chai K. Lim, Martin Samuelsson, Lil Träskman-Bendz, Gilles J. Guillemin, Sophie Erhardt, and Lena Brundin. "A Role for Inflammatory Metabolites as Modulators of the Glutamate N-Methyl-d-Aspartate Receptor in Depression and Suicidality." *Brain, Behavior, and Immunity* 43 (January 2015): 110–17. doi:10.1016/j .bbi.2014.07.012.

Bellisle, France. "Glutamate and the UMAMI Taste: Sensory, Metabolic, Nutritional and Behavioural Considerations. A Review of the Literature Published in the Last 10 Years." *Neuroscience & Biobehavioral Reviews* 23, no. 3 (January 1, 1999): 423–38. doi:10.1016/S0149-7634(98)00043-8.

Bernardinelli, Yann, Irina Nikonenko, and Dominique Muller. "Structural Plasticity: Mechanisms and Contribution to Developmental Psychiatric Disorders." *Frontiers in Neuroanatomy* 8 (November 3, 2014): 123. doi:10.3389/fnana.2014.00123.

Blackshaw, L. A., S. J. H. Brookes, D. Grundy, and M. Schemann. "Sensory Transmission in the Gastrointestinal Tract." *Neurogastroenterology & Motility* 19, no. s1 (January 2007): 1–19. doi:10.1111/j.1365-2982.2006.00871.x.

Blandini, F., and J. T. Greenamyre. "Prospects of Glutamate Antagonists in the Therapy of Parkinson's Disease." *Fundamental & Clinical Pharmacology* 12, no. 1 (January 2, 1998): 4–12. doi:10.1111/j.1472-8206.1998.tb00918.x.

Blandini, Fabio, and Marie-Therese Armentero. "New Pharmacological Avenues for the Treatment of L-dopa-Induced Dyskinesias in Parkinson's Disease: Targeting Glutamate and Adenosine Receptors." *Expert Opinion on Investigational Drugs* 21, no. 2 (January 11, 2012): 153–68. doi:10.1517/13543784.2012.651457.

Blaylock, R., and A. Strunecka. "Immune-Glutamatergic Dysfunction as a Central Mechanism of the Autism Spectrum Disorders." *Current Medicinal Chemistry* 16, no. 2 (January 1, 2009): 157–70. doi:10.2174/092986709787002745.

Blaylock, Russell L. *Excitotoxins: The Taste That Kills.* Santa Fe, NM: Health Press, 1998.

Blaylock, Russell L. *Multiple Sclerosis.* Atlanta, GA: Pritchett & Hull, 1988.

Bolton, Christopher, and Carolyn Paul. "Glutamate Receptors in Neuroinflammatory Demyelinating Disease." *Mediators of Inflammation* 2006 (2006): 1–12. doi:10.1155/mi/2006/93684.

Bonaccio, Marialaura, Augusto Di Castelnuovo, Emilia Ruggiero, Simona Costanzo, Giuseppe Grosso, Amalia De Curtis, Chiara Cerletti, Maria Benedetta Donati, Giovanni de Gaetano, and Licia Iacoviello. "Joint Association of Food Nutritional Profile by Nutri-Score Front-of-Pack Label and Ultra-Processed Food Intake with Mortality: Moli-Sani Prospective Cohort Study." *BMJ* 378 (August 31, 2022): e070688. doi:10.1136/bmj-2022-070688.

Bontemps-Gallo, Sébastien, Kevin Lawrence, and Frank C. Gherardini. "Two Different Virulence-Related Regulatory Pathways in Borrelia Burgdorferi Are Directly Affected by Osmotic Fluxes in the Blood Meal of Feeding

Ixodes Ticks." *PLoS Pathogens* 12, no. 8 (August 15, 2016): e1005791. doi:10.1371/journal.ppat.1005791.

Briguglio, Matteo, Bernardo Dell'Osso, Giancarlo Panzica, Antonio Malgaroli, Giuseppe Banfi, Carlotta Zanaboni Dina, Roberta Galentino, and Mauro Porta. "Dietary Neurotransmitters: A Narrative Review on Current Knowledge." *Nutrients* 10, no. 5 (May 10, 2018): 591. doi:10.3390/nu10050591.

Brown, Mark S., Debra Singel, Susan Hepburn, and Donald C. Rojas. "Increased Glutamate Concentration in the Auditory Cortex of Persons with Autism and First-Degree Relatives: A1H-MRS Study." *Autism Research* 6, no. 1 (November 16, 2012): 1–10. doi:10.1002/aur.1260.

Buck, Silas A., Mary M. Torregrossa, Ryan W. Logan, and Zachary Freyberg. "Roles of Dopamine and Glutamate Co-Release in the Nucleus Accumbens in Mediating the Actions of Drugs of Abuse." *The FEBS Journal* 288, no. 5 (August 11, 2020): 1462–74. doi:10.1111/febs.15496.

Bursey, R. G., L. Watson, and M. Smriga. "A Lack of Epidemiologic Evidence to Link Consumption of Monosodium L-Glutamate and Obesity in China." *American Journal of Clinical Nutrition* 94, no. 3 (August 19, 2011): 958–60. doi:10.3945/ajcn.111.020727.

Cabarrocas, Julie, Tor C. Savidge, and Roland S. Liblau. "Role of Enteric Glial Cells in Inflammatory Bowel Disease." *Glia* 41, no. 1 (December 3, 2002): 81–93. doi:10.1002/glia.10169.

Cahalan, Susannah. *Brain on Fire.* New York: Simon and Schuster, 2013.

Carlson, Greg C. "Glutamate Receptor Dysfunction and Drug Targets across Models of Autism Spectrum Disorders." *Pharmacology Biochemistry and Behavior* 100, no. 4 (February 2012): 850–54. doi:10.1016/j.pbb.2011.02.003.

Cartmell, Jayne, and Darryle D. Schoepp. "Regulation of Neurotransmitter Release by Metabotropic Glutamate Receptors." *Journal of Neurochemistry* 75, no. 3 (January 4, 2002): 889–907. doi:10.1046/j.1471-4159.2000.0750889.x.

Centers for Disease Control and Prevention. "Adult Obesity Facts." February 11, 2021. https://www.cdc.gov/obesity/data/adult.html.

Centers for Disease Control and Prevention. "Alzheimer's Disease and Related Dementias." October 26, 2020. https://www.cdc.gov/aging/aginginfo/alzheimers.htm.

Centers for Disease Control and Prevention. "Data and Statistics about ADHD. September 23, 2021. https://www.cdc.gov/ncbddd/adhd/data.html.

Centers for Disease Control and Prevention. "Data & Statistics on Autism Spectrum Disorder." December 2, 2021. https://www.cdc.gov/ncbddd/autism/data.html.

Centers for Disease Control and Prevention. "Drug Overdose Deaths in the U.S. Top 100,000 Annually." November 17, 2021. https://www.cdc.gov/nchs/pressroom/nchs_press_releases/2021/20211117.htm.

Centers for Disease Control and Prevention. "FastStats: Overweight Prevalence." 2019. https://www.cdc.gov/nchs/fastats/obesity-overweight.htm.

Centers for Disease Control and Prevention. "Health Policy Data Requests—Percent of U.S. Adults 55 and over with Chronic Conditions." 2020. https://www.cdc.gov/nchs/health_policy/adult_chronic_conditions.htm.

Centers for Disease Control and Prevention. "National Diabetes Statistics Report, 2017 Estimates of Diabetes and Its Burden in the United States Background." 2020. https://www.cdc.gov/diabetes/pdfs/data/statistics/national-diabetes-statistics-report.pdf.

Centers for Disease Control and Prevention. "National DPP Customer Service Center." 2022. https://nationaldppcsc.cdc.gov/s/article/CDC-2022-National-Diabetes-Statistics-Report.

Chapman, Astrid G. "Glutamate and Epilepsy." *Journal of Nutrition* 130, no. 4 (April 1, 2000): 1043S1045S. doi:10.1093/jn/130.4.1043s.

Chen, Xiaojia, Zhang Zhang, Huijie Yang, Peishan Qiu, Haizhou Wang, Fan Wang, Qiu Zhao, Jun Fang, and Jiayan Nie. "Consumption of Ultra-Processed Foods and Health Outcomes: A Systematic Review of Epidemiological Studies." *Nutrition Journal* 19, no. 1 (August 20, 2020). doi:10.1186/s12937-020-00604-1.

Choudhury, Paromita Roy, Sanjukta Lahiri, and Usha Rajamma. "Glutamate Mediated Signaling in the Pathophysiology of Autism Spectrum Disorders." *Pharmacology Biochemistry and Behavior* 100, no. 4 (February 2012): 841–49. doi:10.1016/j.pbb.2011.06.023.

Collison, Kate S., Zakia M. Maqbool, Angela L. Inglis, Nadine J. Makhoul, Soad M. Saleh, Razan H. Bakheet, Mohammed A. Al-Johi, Rana K. Al-Rabiah, Marya Z. Zaidi, and Futwan A. Al-Mohanna. "Effect of Dietary Monosodium Glutamate on HFCS-Induced Hepatic Steatosis: Expression Profiles in the Liver and Visceral Fat." *Obesity* 18, no. 6 (June 2010): 1122–34. doi:10.1038/oby.2009.502.

Conlon, Michael, and Anthony Bird. "The Impact of Diet and Lifestyle on Gut Microbiota and Human Health." *Nutrients* 7, no. 1 (December 24, 2014): 17–44. doi:10.3390/nu7010017.

Connolly, Niamh M. C., and Jochen H. M. Prehn. "The Metabolic Response to Excitotoxicity: Lessons from Single-Cell Imaging." *Journal of Bioenergetics and Biomembranes* 47, no. 1–2 (September 28, 2014): 75–88. doi:10.1007/s10863-014-9578-4.

Cornet, Anne, Tor C. Savidge, Julie Cabarrocas, Wen-Lin Deng, Jean-Frederic Colombel, Hans Lassmann, Pierre Desreumaux, and Roland S. Liblau. "Enterocolitis Induced by Autoimmune Targeting of Enteric Glial Cells: A Possible Mechanism in Crohn's Disease?" *Proceedings of the National Academy of Sciences of the United States of America* 98, no. 23 (November 6, 2001): 13306–11. doi:10.1073/pnas.231474098.

Cryan, J. F., and S. M. O'Mahony. "The Microbiome–Gut–Brain Axis: From Bowel to Behavior." *Neurogastroenterology & Motility* 23, no. 3 (February 8, 2011): 187–92. doi:10.1111/j.1365-2982.2010.01664.x.

Cuomo, Dario, Giuseppina Martella, Emanuela Barabino, Paola Platania, Daniela Vita, Graziella Madeo, Chelliah Selvam, et al. "Metabotropic Glutamate Receptor Subtype 4 Selectively Modulates Both Glutamate and GABA Transmission in the Striatum: Implications for Parkinson's Disease Treatment." *Journal of Neurochemistry* 109, no. 4 (May 2009): 1096–1105. doi:10.1111/j.1471-4159.2009.06036.x.

Dantzer, Robert, and Adam K. Walker. "Is There a Role for Glutamate-Mediated Excitotoxicity in Inflammation-Induced Depression?" *Journal of Neural Transmission* 121, no. 8 (March 15, 2014): 925–32. doi:10.1007/s00702-014-1187-1.

Davalli, Alberto M., Carla Perego, and Franco B. Folli. "The Potential Role of Glutamate in the Current Diabetes Epidemic." *Acta Diabetologica* 49, no. 3 (January 5, 2012): 167–83. doi:10.1007/s00592-011-0364-z.

David, Lawrence A., Corinne F. Maurice, Rachel N. Carmody, David B. Gootenberg, Julie E. Button, Benjamin E. Wolfe, Alisha V. Ling, et al. "Diet Rapidly and Reproducibly Alters the Human Gut Microbiome." *Nature* 505, no. 7484 (December 11, 2013): 559–63. doi:10.1038/nature12820.

De Filippo, C., D. Cavalieri, M. Di Paola, M. Ramazzotti, J. B. Poullet, S. Massart, S. Collini, G. Pieraccini, and P. Lionetti. "Impact of Diet in Shaping Gut Microbiota Revealed by a Comparative Study in Children from Europe and Rural Africa." *Proceedings of the National Academy of Sciences* 107, no. 33 (August 2, 2010): 14691–96. doi:10.1073/pnas.1005963107.

De Wandel, Sofie, Marielle P. K. J. Engelen, Raven Wierzchowska-McNew, Julie Thompson, Sarah K. Kirschner, Clayton L. Cruthirds, Gabriella A. M. Ten Have, John J. Thaden, and Nicolaas E. P. Deutz. "Altered Glutamate and Glutamine Kinetics in Autism Spectrum Disorder." *Current Developments in Nutrition* 5, no. Supplement, 2 (June 2021): 845–45. doi:10.1093/cdn/nzab047_008.

Derkach, Victor A., Michael C. Oh, Eric S. Guire, and Thomas R. Soderling. "Regulatory Mechanisms of AMPA Receptors in Synaptic Plasticity."

Nature Reviews Neuroscience 8, no. 2 (February 2007): 101–13. doi:10.1038 /nrn2055.

Dogtor J. "DogtorJ.com: Food Intolerance in Pets & Their People: Home of the GARD." 2009. https://dogtorj.com.

Doidge, Norman. *The Brain That Changes Itself: Stories of Personal Triumph from the Frontiers of Brain Science.* Melbourne: Scribe, 2007.

Dukowicz, Andrew C., Brian E. Lacy, and Gary M. Levine. "Small Intestinal Bacterial Overgrowth: A Comprehensive Review." *Gastroenterology & Hepatology* 3, no. 2 (February 1, 2007): 112–22. https://www.ncbi.nlm.nih .gov/pubmed/21960820.

Eggermont, Jos. J., and Larry E. Roberts. "The Neuroscience of Tinnitus: Understanding Abnormal and Normal Auditory Perception." *Frontiers in Systems Neuroscience* 6 (2012). doi:10.3389/fnsys.2012.00053.

El-Ansary, A. "GABA and Glutamate Imbalance in Autism and Their Reversal as Novel Hypothesis for Effective Treatment Strategy." *Autism and Developmental Disorders* 18, no. 3 (2020): 46–63. doi:10.17759/aut dd.2020180306.

Ende, Gabriele, Sylvia Cackowski, Julia Van Eijk, Markus Sack, Traute Demirakca, Nikolaus Kleindienst, Martin Bohus, Esther Sobanski, Annegret Krause-Utz, and Christian Schmahl. "Impulsivity and Aggression in Female BPD and ADHD Patients: Association with ACC Glutamate and GABA Concentrations." *Neuropsychopharmacology* 41, no. 2 (June 4, 2015): 410–18. doi:10.1038/npp.2015.153.

Erb, John. "Revoke the GRAS Standing of the Food Additive Monosodium Glutamate." Citizens Petition FDA-2007-P-0178-0002. Food and Drug Administration," 2008.

Erb, John E., and T. Michelle Erb. *The Slow Poisoning of America.* Virginia Beach, VA: Paladins Press, 2003.

Erdozain, Amaia M., and Luis F. Callado. "Neurobiological Alterations in Alcohol Addiction: A Review." *Adicciones* 26, no. 4 (2014): 360–70. http:// www.ncbi.nlm.nih.gov/pubmed/25578004.

Essa, M. M., N. Braidy, K. R. Vijayan, S. Subash, and G. J. Guillemin. "Excitotoxity in the Pathogenesis of Autism." *Neurotoxicity Research* 23, no. 4 (October 13, 2012): 393–400. doi:10.1007/s12640-012-9354-3.

Faith, J. J., N. P. McNulty, F. E. Rey, and J. I. Gordon. "Predicting a Human Gut Microbiota's Response to Diet in Gnotobiotic Mice." *Science* 333, no. 6038 (May 19, 2011): 101–4. doi:10.1126/science.1206025.

FDA Letters. "You Have the Right to Know What Is in Your Food." Citizens Petition # 94P-0444. U.S. Food and Drug Administration. Department of Health and Human Services. September 15, 1995.

Feng, Ze-Meng, Tie-Jun Li, Li Wu, Ding-Fu Xiao, Francois Blachier, and Yulong Yin. "Monosodium L-Glutamate and Dietary Fat Differently Modify the Composition of the Intestinal Microbiota in Growing Pigs." *Obesity Facts* 8, no. 2 (2015): 87–100. doi:10.1159/000380889.

Feng, Zemeng, Tiejun Li, Chunli Wu, Lihua Tao, Francois Blachier, and Yulong Yin. "Monosodium L-Glutamate and Dietary Fat Exert Opposite Effects on the Proximal and Distal Intestinal Health in Growing Pigs." *Applied Physiology, Nutrition, and Metabolism* 40, no. 4 (April 2015): 353–63. doi:10.1139/apnm-2014-0434.

Fernandez-Tresguerres Hernández, Jesus A. "Effect of Monosodium Glutamate Given Orally on Appetite Control (a New Theory for the Obesity Epidemic)." *Anales de La Real Academia Nacional de Medicina* 122, no. 2 (2005): 341–55; discussion 355–360. http://www.ncbi.nlm.nih.gov/pubmed/16463577.

Filippi, Massimo, Maria A. Rocca, Frederik Barkhof, Wolfgang Brück, Jacqueline T. Chen, Giancarlo Comi, Gabriele DeLuca, et al. "Association between Pathological and MRI Findings in Multiple Sclerosis." *The Lancet Neurology* 11, no. 4 (April 2012): 349–60. doi:10.1016/s1474-4422(12)70003-0.

Filpa, Viviana, Elisabetta Moro, Marina Protasoni, Francesca Crema, Gianmario Frigo, and Cristina Giaroni. "Role of Glutamatergic Neurotransmission in the Enteric Nervous System and Brain-Gut Axis in Health and Disease." *Neuropharmacology* 111 (December 2016): 14–33. doi:10.1016/j.neuropharm.2016.08.024.

Finkel, Alan G., Juanita A. Yerry, and J. Douglas Mann. "Dietary Considerations in Migraine Management: Does a Consistent Diet Improve Migraine?" *Current Pain and Headache Reports* 17, no. 11 (September 26, 2013). doi:10.1007/s11916-013-0373-4.

Fooducate. "No Product Found." Accessed December 8, 2022. https://www.fooducate.com/product/KFC-Chicken-Pot-Pie/8963DD6E-398F-11E3-A74D-1E047F0525AB.

Friedberg, M., B. Saffran, T. J. Stinson, W. Nelson, and C. L. Bennett. "Evaluation of Conflict of Interest in Economic Analyses of New Drugs Used in Oncology." *JAMA* 282, no. 15 (October 20, 1999): 1453–57. doi:10.1001/jama.282.15.1453.

Fujimoto, Makoto, Koichi Tsuneyama, Yuko Nakanishi, Thucydides L. Salunga, Kazuhiro Nomoto, Yoshiyuki Sasaki, Seiichi Iizuka, et al. "A Dietary Restriction Influences the Progression but Not the Initiation of MSG-Induced Nonalcoholic Steatohepatitis." *Journal of Medicinal Food* 17, no. 3 (March 2014): 374–83. doi:10.1089/jmf.2012.0029.

Gao, Lu, Tiansong Xu, Gang Huang, Song Jiang, Yan Gu, and Feng Chen. "Oral Microbiomes: More and More Importance in Oral Cavity and Whole Body." *Protein & Cell* 9, no. 5 (May 2018): 488–500. doi:10.1007 /s13238-018-0548-1.

Gentile, Christopher L., and Tiffany L. Weir. "The Gut Microbiota at the Intersection of Diet and Human Health." *Science* 362, no. 6416 (November 15, 2018): 776–80. doi:10.1126/science.aau5812.

Gobatto, C. A., M. a. R. Mello, C. T. Souza, and I. A. Ribeiro. "The Monosodium Glutamate (MSG) Obese Rat as a Model for the Study of Exercise in Obesity." *Research Communications in Molecular Pathology and Pharmacology* 111, no. 1–4 (2002): 89–101. http://www.ncbi.nlm.nih.gov /pubmed/14632317.

Grubišić, Vladimir, Alexei Verkhratsky, Robert Zorec, and Vladimir Parpura. "Enteric Glia Regulate Gut Motility in Health and Disease." *Brain Research Bulletin* 136 (January 2018): 109–17. doi:10.1016/j .brainresbull.2017.03.011.

Gupta, Arpana, Vadim Osadchiy, and Emeran A. Mayer. "Brain–Gut–Microbiome Interactions in Obesity and Food Addiction." *Nature Reviews Gastroenterology & Hepatology* 17, no. 11 (August 27, 2020): 655–72. doi:10.1038/s41575-020-0341-5.

Hall, Kevin D., Alexis Ayuketah, Robert Brychta, Hongyi Cai, Thomas Cassimatis, Kong Y. Chen, Stephanie T. Chung, et al. "Ultra-Processed Diets Cause Excess Calorie Intake and Weight Gain: An Inpatient Randomized Controlled Trial of Ad Libitum Food Intake." *Cell Metabolism* 30, no. 1 (July 2019): 226. doi:10.1016/j.cmet.2019.05.020.

Hammit, L. "Glutamate Identified as Predictor of Disease Progression in Multiple Sclerosis." University of California San Francisco, April 29, 2009. https://www.ucsf.edu/news/2009/04/4227/glutamate-identified-predictor -disease-progression-multiple-sclero.

Hansen, Anna M., and Rachel R. Caspi. "Glutamate Joins the Ranks of Immunomodulators." *Nature Medicine* 16, no. 8 (August 2010): 856–58. doi:10.1038/nm0810-856.

Haroon, Ebrahim, Andrew H. Miller, and Gerard Sanacora. "Inflammation, Glutamate, and Glia: A Trio of Trouble in Mood Disorders." *Neuropsychopharmacology* 42, no. 1 (September 15, 2016): 193–215. doi:10.1038/npp.2016.199.

Hashimoto, Kenji, Akira Sawa, and Masaomi Iyo. "Increased Levels of Glutamate in Brains from Patients with Mood Disorders." *Biological Psychiatry* 62, no. 11 (December 2007): 1310–16. doi:10.1016/j.biopsych.2007.03.017.

He, Ka, Shufa Du, Pengcheng Xun, Sangita Sharma, Huijun Wang, Fengying Zhai, and Barry Popkin. "Consumption of Monosodium Glutamate in Relation to Incidence of Overweight in Chinese Adults: China Health and Nutrition Survey (CHNS)." *American Journal of Clinical Nutrition* 93, no. 6 (April 6, 2011): 1328–36. doi:10.3945/ajcn.110.008870.

Helms, Hans Christian, Rasmus Madelung, Helle Sønderby Waagepetersen, Carsten Uhd Nielsen, and Birger Brodin. "In Vitro Evidence for the Brain Glutamate Efflux Hypothesis: Brain Endothelial Cells Cocultured with Astrocytes Display a Polarized Brain-To-Blood Transport of Glutamate." *Glia* 60, no. 6 (March 5, 2012): 882–93. doi:10.1002/glia.22321.

Herbert, Martha R., and Karen Weintraub. *The Autism Revolution: Whole-Body Strategies for Making Life All It Can Be*. New York: Ballantine Books, 2012.

Herman, Barbara H. *Glutamate and Addiction*. Springer Science & Business Media, 2002.

Hermanussen, M., A. P. García, M. Sunder, M. Voigt, V. Salazar, and J. A. F. Tresguerres. "Obesity, Voracity, and Short Stature: The Impact of Glutamate on the Regulation of Appetite." *European Journal of Clinical Nutrition* 60, no. 1 (August 31, 2005): 25–31. doi:10.1038/sj.ejcn.1602263.

Hirata, A. E., I. S. Andrade, P. Vaskevicius, and M. S. Dolnikoff. "Monosodium Glutamate (MSG)-Obese Rats Develop Glucose Intolerance and Insulin Resistance to Peripheral Glucose Uptake." *Brazilian Journal of Medical and Biological Research* 30, no. 5 (May 1997): 671–667. doi:10.1590/s0100-879x1997000500016.

Holmes, Elaine, Jia V. Li, Thanos Athanasiou, Hutan Ashrafian, and Jeremy K. Nicholson. "Understanding the Role of Gut Microbiome–Host Metabolic Signal Disruption in Health and Disease." *Trends in Microbiology* 19, no. 7 (July 2011): 349–59. doi:10.1016/j.tim.2011.05.006.

Holmes, Sophie E., Matthew J. Girgenti, Margaret T. Davis, Robert H. Pietrzak, Nicole DellaGioia, Nabeel Nabulsi, David Matuskey, et al. "Altered Metabotropic Glutamate Receptor 5 Markers in PTSD: In Vivo and Postmortem Evidence." *Proceedings of the National Academy of Sciences*, July 12, 2017. doi:10.1073/pnas.1701749114.

Holton, Kathleen F., Peter K. Ndege, and Daniel J. Clauw. "Dietary Correlates of Chronic Widespread Pain in Meru, Kenya." *Nutrition* 53 (September 2018): 14–19. doi:10.1016/j.nut.2018.01.016.

Holton, Kathleen Feeney, Douglas L. Taren, Robert M. Bennett, and Kim Dupree Jones. "Novel Dietary Intervention Produces Significant Improvements in Fibromyalgia Patients with Irritable Bowel Syndrome." *FASEB Journal* 24, no. S1 (April 2010).

Hooper, L. V. "Molecular Analysis of Commensal Host-Microbial Relationships in the Intestine." *Science* 291, no. 5505 (February 2, 2001): 881–84. doi:10.1126/science.291.5505.881.

Hughes, R., E. A. Magee, and S. Bingham. "Protein Degradation in the Large Intestine: Relevance to Colorectal Cancer." *Current Issues in Intestinal Microbiology* 1, no. 2 (September 1, 2000): 51–58. http://www.ncbi.nlm.nih.gov/pubmed/11709869.

Hyman, Mark. *The UltraMind Solution: Fix Your Broken Brain by Healing Your Body First: The Simple Way to Defeat Depression, Overcome Anxiety, and Sharpen Your Mind.* New York: Scribner, 2009.

Hynd, M. "Glutamate-Mediated Excitotoxicity and Neurodegeneration in Alzheimer's Disease." *Neurochemistry International* 45, no. 5 (October 2004): 583–95. doi:10.1016/j.neuint.2004.03.007.

Iati, Marisa. "He Was Acting Drunk but Swore He Was Sober. Turns out His Stomach Was Brewing Its Own Beer." *Washington Post*, October 30, 2019. https://www.washingtonpost.com/health/2019/10/24/he-was-acting-drunk-swore-he-was-sober-turns-out-his-stomach-was-brewing-its-own-beer/.

Insawang, Tonkla, Carlo Selmi, Ubon Cha'on, Supattra Pethlert, Puangrat Yongvanit, Premjai Areejitranusorn, Patcharee Boonsiri, et al. "Monosodium Glutamate (MSG) Intake Is Associated with the Prevalence of Metabolic Syndrome in a Rural Thai Population." *Nutrition & Metabolism* 9, no. 1 (2012): 50. doi:10.1186/1743-7075-9-50.

International Food Information Council. "Everything You Need to Know about Glutamate and Monosodium Glutamate." Food Insight, October 17, 2009. https://foodinsight.org/everything-you-need-to-know-about-glutamate-and-monosodium-glutamate.

Islam, M. S., and D. T. Loots. "Experimental Rodent Models of Type 2 Diabetes: A Review." *Methods and Findings in Experimental and Clinical Pharmacology* 31, no. 4 (2009): 249. doi:10.1358/mf.2009.31.4.1362513.

Ivens, S., D. Kaufer, L. P. Flores, I. Bechmann, D. Zumsteg, O. Tomkins, E. Seiffert, U. Heinemann, and A. Friedman. "TGF-beta Receptor-Mediated Albumin Uptake into Astrocytes Is Involved in Neocortical Epileptogenesis." *Brain* 130, no. 2 (February 1, 2007): 535–47. doi:10.1093/brain/awl317.

Janssen, Raelyn, Laura Schweitzer, and Karl F. Jensen. "Glutamate Neurotoxicity in the Developing Rat Cochlea: Physiological and Morphological Approaches." *Brain Research* 552, no. 2 (June 1991): 255–64. doi:10.1016/0006-8993(91)90090-i.

Jeon, Peter, Roberto Limongi, Sabrina D. Ford, Michael Mackinley, Kara Dempster, Jean Théberge, and Lena Palaniyappan. "Progressive Changes in Glutamate Concentration in Early Stages of Schizophrenia: A Longitudinal 7-Tesla MRS Study." *Schizophrenia Bulletin Open* 2, no. 1 (January 1, 2021). doi:10.1093/schizbullopen/sgaa072.

Jiang, Shu-Heng, Li-Peng Hu, Xu Wang, Jun Li, and Zhi-Gang Zhang. "Neurotransmitters: Emerging Targets in Cancer." *Oncogene* 39, no. 3 (September 16, 2019): 503–15. doi:10.1038/s41388-019-1006-0.

Johns Hopkins Medicine. "Mental Health Disorder Statistics." 2019. https://www.hopkinsmedicine.org/health/wellness-and-prevention/mental-health-disorder-statistics.

Julio-Pieper, Marcela, Peter J. Flor, Timothy G. Dinan, and John F. Cryan. "Exciting Times beyond the Brain: Metabotropic Glutamate Receptors in Peripheral and Non-Neural Tissues." *Pharmacological Reviews* 63, no. 1 (January 12, 2011): 35–58. doi:10.1124/pr.110.004036.

Kalivas, P. "Glutamate Systems in Cocaine Addiction." *Current Opinion in Pharmacology* 4, no. 1 (February 2004): 23–29. doi:10.1016/j.coph.2003.11.002.

Kanarek, Robin B., Julie Meyers, Robert G. Meade, and Jean Mayer. "Juvenile-Onset Obesity and Deficits in Caloric Regulation in MSG-Treated Rats." *Pharmacology Biochemistry and Behavior* 10, no. 5 (May 1979): 717–21. doi:10.1016/0091-3057(79)90324-1.

Kang, Dae-Wook, James B. Adams, Devon M. Coleman, Elena L. Pollard, Juan Maldonado, Sharon McDonough-Means, J. Gregory Caporaso, and Rosa Krajmalnik-Brown. "Long-Term Benefit of Microbiota Transfer Therapy on Autism Symptoms and Gut Microbiota." *Scientific Reports* 9, no. 1 (April 9, 2019). doi:10.1038/s41598-019-42183-0.

Karin, Michael, Toby Lawrence, and Victor Nizet. "Innate Immunity Gone Awry: Linking Microbial Infections to Chronic Inflammation and Cancer." *Cell* 124, no. 4 (February 2006): 823–35. doi:10.1016/j.cell.2006.02.016.

Kawase, Takahiro, Mao Nagasawa, Hiromi Ikeda, Shinobu Yasuo, Yasuhiro Koga, and Mitsuhiro Furuse. "Gut Microbiota of Mice Putatively Modifies Amino Acid Metabolism in the Host Brain." *British Journal of Nutrition* 117, no. 6 (March 1, 2017): 775–83. doi:10.1017/S0007114517000678.

Khairunnisak, M., A. H. Azizah, S. Jinap, and A. Nurul Izzah. "Monitoring of Free Glutamic Acid in Malaysian Processed Foods, Dishes and Condiments." *Food Additives & Contaminants: Part A* 26, no. 4 (April 2009): 419–26. doi:10.1080/02652030802596860.

Khandaker, Golam M., and Robert Dantzer. "Is There a Role for Immune-To-Brain Communication in Schizophrenia?" *Psychopharmacology* 233, no. 9 (June 4, 2015): 1559–73. doi:10.1007/s00213-015-3975-1.

Kirchgessner, Annette L., Min-Tsai Liu, and Frederick Alcantara. "Excitotoxicity in the Enteric Nervous System." *Journal of Neuroscience* 17, no. 22 (November 15, 1997): 8804–16. doi:10.1523/jneurosci.17-22-08804.1997.

Labus, Jennifer S., Vadim Osadchiy, Elaine Y. Hsiao, Julien Tap, Muriel Derrien, Arpana Gupta, Kirsten Tillisch, et al. "Evidence for an Association of Gut Microbial Clostridia with Brain Functional Connectivity and Gastrointestinal Sensorimotor Function in Patients with Irritable Bowel Syndrome, Based on Tripartite Network Analysis." *Microbiome* 7, no. 1 (March 21, 2019). doi:10.1186/s40168-019-0656-z.

Lachance, Laura R., and Kwame McKenzie. "Biomarkers of Gluten Sensitivity in Patients with Non-Affective Psychosis: A Meta-Analysis." *Schizophrenia Research* 152, no. 2–3 (February 2014): 521–27. doi:10.1016/j.schres.2013.12.001.

Lai, Kwok-On, and Nancy Y. Ip. "Structural Plasticity of Dendritic Spines: The Underlying Mechanisms and Its Dysregulation in Brain Disorders." *Biochimica et Biophysica Acta (BBA)—Molecular Basis of Disease* 1832, no. 12 (December 1, 2013): 2257–63. doi:10.1016/j.bbadis.2013.08.012.

Landa, Michael. "FDA/CFSAN to John Erb—Petition Denial. FDA-2007-P-0178. U.S. Food and Drug Administration, Health and Human Services, 2012.

Lee, Hyoung-gon, Xiongwei Zhu, Michael J. O'Neill, Kate Webber, Gemma Casadesus, Michael Marlatt, Arun K. Raina, George Perry, and Mark A. Smith. "The Role of Metabotropic Glutamate Receptors in Alzheimer's Disease." *Acta Neurobiologiae Experimentalis* 64, no. 1 (2004): 89–98. http://www.ncbi.nlm.nih.gov/pubmed/15190683.

Lexchin, J. "Pharmaceutical Industry Sponsorship and Research Outcome and Quality: Systematic Review." *BMJ* 326, no. 7400 (May 29, 2003): 1167–70. doi:10.1136/bmj.326.7400.1167.

Liu, Min-Tsai, Jeffrey D. Rothstein, Michael D. Gershon, and Annette L. Kirchgessner. "Glutamatergic Enteric Neurons." *Journal of Neuroscience* 17, no. 12 (June 15, 1997): 4764–84. doi:10.1523/jneurosci.17-12-04764.1997.

Liu, Ruixin, Jie Hong, Xiaoqiang Xu, Qiang Feng, Dongya Zhang, Yanyun Gu, Juan Shi, et al. "Gut Microbiome and Serum Metabolome Alterations in Obesity and after Weight-Loss Intervention." *Nature Medicine* 23, no. 7 (June 19, 2017): 859–68. doi:10.1038/nm.4358.

Longoni, M., and C. Ferrarese. "Inflammation and Excitotoxicity: Role in Migraine Pathogenesis." *Neurological Sciences* 27, no. S2 (May 2006): s107–10. doi:10.1007/s10072-006-0582-2.

Lucas, D. R., and J. P. Newhouse. "The Toxic Effect of Sodium L-Glutamate on the Inner Layers of the Retina." *Archives of Ophthalmology* 58, no. 2 (August 1, 1957): 193–201. doi:10.1001/archopht.1957.00940010205006.

Lumpkin, Ellen A., and Michael J. Caterina. "Mechanisms of Sensory Transduction in the Skin." *Nature* 445, no. 7130 (February 2007): 858–65. doi:10.1038/nature05662.

Luna, Ruth Ann, and Jane A. Foster. "Gut Brain Axis: Diet Microbiota Interactions and Implications for Modulation of Anxiety and Depression." *Current Opinion in Biotechnology* 32 (April 2015): 35–41. doi:10.1016/j.copbio.2014.10.007.

Lutas, Andrew, and Gary Yellen. "The Ketogenic Diet: Metabolic Influences on Brain Excitability and Epilepsy." *Trends in Neurosciences* 36, no. 1 (January 2013): 32–40. doi:10.1016/j.tins.2012.11.005.

Macho, L., M. Ficková, D. Jezová, and S. Zórad. "Late Effects of Postnatal Administration of Monosodium Glutamate on Insulin Action in Adult Rats." *Physiological Research* 49, Supplement 1 (2000): S79–85. http://www.ncbi.nlm.nih.gov/pubmed/10984075.

MacIntyre, Angela, Christine J. Hammond, C. Scott Little, Denah M. Appelt, and Brian J. Balin. "*Chlamydia Pneumoniae* Infection Alters the Junctional Complex Proteins of Human Brain Microvascular Endothelial Cells." *FEMS Microbiology Letters* 217, no. 2 (December 2002): 167–72. doi:10.1111/j.1574-6968.2002.tb11470.x.

Macrez, Richard, Peter K. Stys, Denis Vivien, Stuart A. Lipton, and Fabian Docagne. "Mechanisms of Glutamate Toxicity in Multiple Sclerosis: Biomarker and Therapeutic Opportunities." *The Lancet Neurology* 15, no. 10 (September 2016): 1089–1102. doi:10.1016/s1474-4422(16)30165-x.

Maia Research Co., Ltd. "Global Monosodium Glutamate Production and Consumption from 2021–2022." 2022.

Maragos, William F., J. Timothy Greenamyre, John B. Penney, and Anne B. Young. "Glutamate Dysfunction in Alzheimer's Disease: An Hypothesis." *Trends in Neurosciences* 10, no. 2 (February 1987): 65–68. doi:10.1016/0166-2236(87)90025-7.

Martínez Steele, Eurídice, Larissa Galastri Baraldi, Maria Laura da Costa Louzada, Jean-Claude Moubarac, Dariush Mozaffarian, and Carlos Augusto Monteiro. "Ultra-Processed Foods and Added Sugars in the US Diet: Evidence from a Nationally Representative Cross-Sectional

Study." *BMJ Open* 6, no. 3 (January 2016): e009892. doi:10.1136/bmjopen -2015-009892.

Matsumoto, Mitsuharu, Ryoko Kibe, Takushi Ooga, Yuji Aiba, Emiko Sawaki, Yasuhiro Koga, and Yoshimi Benno. "Cerebral Low-Molecular Metabolites Influenced by Intestinal Microbiota: A Pilot Study." *Frontiers in Systems Neuroscience* 7 (2013). doi:10.3389/fnsys.2013.00009.

Mayer, Emeran A., Kirsten Tillisch, and Arpana Gupta. "Gut/Brain Axis and the Microbiota." *Journal of Clinical Investigation* 125, no. 3 (February 17, 2015): 926–38. doi:10.1172/jci76304.

McCarthy, Dennis J., Robert Alexander, Mark A. Smith, Sanjeev Pathak, Stephen Kanes, Chi-Ming Lee, and Gerard Sanacora. "Glutamate-Based Depression GBD." *Medical Hypotheses* 78, no. 5 (May 2012): 675–81. doi:10.1016/j.mehy.2012.02.009.

McGrath, Thomas, Richard Baskerville, Marcelo Rogero, and Linda Castell. "Emerging Evidence for the Widespread Role of Glutamatergic Dysfunction in Neuropsychiatric Diseases." *Nutrients* 14, no. 5 (February 22, 2022): 917. doi:10.3390/nu14050917.

McNally, Leah, Zubin Bhagwagar, and Jonas Hannestad. "Inflammation, Glutamate, and Glia in Depression: A Literature Review." *CNS Spectrums* 13, no. 6 (June 1, 2008): 501–10. doi:10.1017/s1092852900016734.

Meldrum, B. "Amino Acids as Dietary Excitotoxins: A Contribution to Understanding Neurodegenerative Disorders." *Brain Research Reviews* 18, no. 3 (December 1993): 293–314. doi:10.1016/0165-0173(93)90014-q.

Mennella, Julie A., Catherine A. Forestell, Lindsay K. Morgan, and Gary K. Beauchamp. "Early Milk Feeding Influences Taste Acceptance and Liking during Infancy." *American Journal of Clinical Nutrition* 90, no. 3 (July 15, 2009): 780S788S. doi:10.3945/ajcn.2009.27462o.

Midtvedt, Tore. "The Gut: A Triggering Place for Autism—Possibilities and Challenges." *Microbial Ecology in Health & Disease* 23 (August 24, 2012). doi:10.3402/mehd.v23i0.18982.

Millichap, J. Gordon, and Michelle M. Yee. "The Diet Factor in Pediatric and Adolescent Migraine." *Pediatric Neurology* 28, no. 1 (January 2003): 9–15. doi:10.1016/s0887-8994(02)00466-6.

Mitani, Hideaki, Yukihiko Shirayama, Takeshi Yamada, Kazuhisa Maeda, Charles R. Ashby, and Ryuzou Kawahara. "Correlation between Plasma Levels of Glutamate, Alanine and Serine with Severity of Depression." *Progress in Neuro-Psychopharmacology and Biological Psychiatry* 30, no. 6 (August 2006): 1155–58. doi:10.1016/j.pnpbp.2006.03.036.

Mohammed, Saher S. "Monosodium Glutamate-Induced Genotoxicity in Rat Palatal Mucosa." *Tanta Dental Journal* 14, no. 3 (2017): 112. Doi:10.4103 /tdj.tdj_20_17.

Monteiro, C. A., J.-C. Moubarac, G. Cannon, S. W. Ng, and B. Popkin. "Ultra-Processed Products Are Becoming Dominant in the Global Food System." *Obesity Reviews* 14 (October 23, 2013): 21–28. Doi:10.1111 /obr.12107.

Monteiro, Carlos Augusto, Geoffrey Cannon, Jean-Claude Moubarac, Renata Bertazzi Levy, Maria Laura C. Louzada, and Patrícia Constante Jaime. "The UN Decade of Nutrition, the NOVA Food Classification and the Trouble with Ultra-Processing." *Public Health Nutrition* 21, no. 1 (March 21, 2017): 5–17. Doi:10.1017/s1368980017000234.

Moss, Michael. "The Extraordinary Science of Addictive Junk Food." *New York Times Magazine*, February 20, 2013. https://www.nytimes.com/2013 /02/24/magazine/the-extraordinary-science-of-junk-food.html.

Most, Dana, Laura Ferguson, and R. Adron Harris. "Molecular Basis of Alcoholism." *Handbook of Clinical Neurology*, 2014, 89–111. doi:10.1016 /b978-0-444-62619-6.00006-9.

Moubarac, Jean-Claude, Ana Paula Bortoletto Martins, Rafael Moreira Claro, Renata Bertazzi Levy, Geoffrey Cannon, and Carlos Augusto Monteiro. "Consumption of Ultra-Processed Foods and Likely Impact on Human Health. Evidence from Canada." *Public Health Nutrition* 16, no. 12 (November 21, 2012): 2240–48. doi:10.1017/s1368980012005009.

Moubarac, Jean-Claude, M. Batal, M. L. Louzada, E. Martinez Steele, and C. A. Monteiro. "Consumption of Ultra-Processed Foods Predicts Diet Quality in Canada." *Appetite* 108 (January 2017): 512–20. doi:10.1016/j .appet.2016.11.006.

Müller, Norbert. "Inflammation and the Glutamate System in Schizophrenia: Implications for Therapeutic Targets and Drug Development." *Expert Opinion on Therapeutic Targets* 12, no. 12 (November 13, 2008): 1497–1507. doi:10.1517/14728220802507852.

Müller, N., and M. J. Schwarz. "The Immune-Mediated Alteration of Serotonin and Glutamate: Towards an Integrated View of Depression." *Molecular Psychiatry* 12, no. 11 (April 24, 2007): 988–1000. doi:10.1038 /sj.mp.4002006.

Nakanishi, Yuko, Koichi Tsuneyama, Makoto Fujimoto, Thucydides L. Salunga, Kazuhiro Nomoto, Jun-Ling An, Yasuo Takano, et al. "Monosodium Glutamate (MSG): A Villain and Promoter of Liver Inflammation and Dysplasia." *Journal of Autoimmunity* 30, no. 1 (February 1, 2008): 42–50. doi:10.1016/j.jaut.2007.11.016.

Nardocci, Milena, Bernard-Simon Leclerc, Maria-Laura Louzada, Carlos Augusto Monteiro, Malek Batal, and Jean-Claude Moubarac. "Consumption of Ultra-Processed Foods and Obesity in Canada." *Canadian Journal of Public Health = Revue Canadienne de Sante Publique* 110, no. 1 (2019): 4–14. doi:10.17269/s41997-018-0130-x.

National Institute on Alcohol Abuse and Alcoholism. "Alcohol Facts and Statistics." March 2022. https://www.niaaa.nih.gov/publications /brochures-and-fact-sheets/alcohol-facts-and-statistics.

NaturalNews.com. "Busted! KFC, Chick-Fil-A, Burger King and Other Fast Food Restaurants Caught Using Huge Quantities of MSG While Calling Their Menu Items Fresh." Accessed December 8, 2022. https://www.nat uralnews.com/KFC-Chick-fil-A-Burger-King-Pizza-Hut-MSG-menu -items.html.

Naviaux, R. K. "Metabolic Features of the Cell Danger Response." *Mitochondrion* 16 (May 1, 2014): 7–17. doi:10.1016/j.mito.2013.08.006.

Neltner, Thomas G., Heather M. Alger, James T. O'Reilly, Sheldon Krimsky, Lisa A. Bero, and Maricel V. Maffini. "Conflicts of Interest in Approvals of Additives to Food Determined to Be Generally Recognized as Safe." *JAMA Internal Medicine* 173, no. 22 (December 9, 2013): 2032. doi:10.1001 /jamainternmed.2013.10559.

Neltner, Thomas G., Neesha R. Kulkarni, Heather M. Alger, Maricel V. Maffini, Erin D. Bongard, Neal D. Fortin, and Erik D. Olson. "Navigating the U.S. Food Additive Regulatory Program." *Comprehensive Reviews in Food Science and Food Safety* 10, no. 6 (October 25, 2011): 342–68. doi:10.1111/j.1541-4337.2011.00166.x.

Nestle, Marion. "Conflicts of Interest in the Regulation of Food Safety." *JAMA Internal Medicine* 173, no. 22 (December 9, 2013): 2036. doi:10.1001 /jamainternmed.2013.9158.

Niijima, Akira. "Reflex Effects of Oral, Gastrointestinal and Hepatoportal Glutamate Sensors on Vagal Nerve Activity." *Journal of Nutrition* 130, no. 4 (April 1, 2000): 971S–973S. doi:10.1093/jn/130.4.971s.

Nilson, Eduardo A. F., Gerson Ferrari, Maria Laura C. Louzada, Renata B. Levy, Carlos A. Monteiro, and Leandro F. M. Rezende. "Premature Deaths Attributable to the Consumption of Ultraprocessed Foods in Brazil." *American Journal of Preventive Medicine* 64, no. 1 (November 7, 2022). doi:10.1016/j.amepre.2022.08.013.

Niro, Serena, Mariantonietta Succi, Patrizio Tremonte, Elena Sorrentino, Raffaele Coppola, Gianfranco Panfili, and Alessandra Fratianni. "Evolution of Free Amino Acids during Ripening of Caciocavallo Cheeses Made with

Different Milks." *Journal of Dairy Science* 100, no. 12 (December 2017): 9521–31. doi:10.3168/jds.2017-13308.

O'Gorman Tuura, Ruth L., Christian R. Baumann, and Heide Baumann-Vogel. "Beyond Dopamine: GABA, Glutamate, and the Axial Symptoms of Parkinson's Disease." *Frontiers in Neurology* 9 (September 26, 2018). doi:10.3389/fneur.2018.00806.

Oliva Ramirez, Abril, Alexander Keenan, Olivia Kalau, Evelyn Worthington, Lucas Cohen, and Sumeet Singh. "Prevalence and Burden of Multiple Sclerosis-Related Fatigue: A Systematic Literature Review." *BMC Neurology* 21, no. 1 (December 2021). doi:10.1186/s12883-021-02396-1.

Olney, J. W. "Brain Lesions, Obesity, and Other Disturbances in Mice Treated with Monosodium Glutamate." *Science (New York, NY)* 164, no. 3880 (1969): 719–21. doi:10.1126/science.164.3880.719.

Olney, J. W. "Excitotoxic Food Additives—Relevance of Animal Studies to Human Safety." *Neurobehavioral Toxicology and Teratology* 6, no. 6 (November 1, 1984): 455–62. http://www.ncbi.nlm.nih.gov/pubmed/6152304.

Olney, J. W. "Excitotoxin-Mediated Neuron Death in Youth and Old Age." *Progress in Brain Research* 86 (1990): 37–51. doi:10.1016/s0079-6123(08)63165-9.

Olney, J. W., and L. G. Sharpe. "Brain Lesions in an Infant Rhesus Monkey Treated with Monosodium Glutamate." *Science* 166, no. 3903 (October 17, 1969): 386–88. doi:10.1126/science.166.3903.386.

Olney, J. W., N. J. Adamo, and A. Ratner. "Monosodium Glutamate Effects." *Science* 172, no. 3980 (April 16, 1971): 294–94. doi:10.1126/science.172.3980.294.

Olney, John W. "Excitatory Amino Acids and Neuropsychiatric Disorders." *Biological Psychiatry* 26, no. 5 (September 1989): 505–25. doi:10.1016/0006-3223(89)90072-3.

Olney, John W. "Excitotoxic Food Additives: Functional Teratological Aspects." *Progress in Brain Research*, 1988, 283–94. doi:10.1016/s0079-6123(08)60510-5.

Olney, John W. "Fetal Alcohol Syndrome at the Cellular Level." *Addiction Biology* 9, no. 2 (June 2004): 137–49. doi:10.1080/13556210410001717006.

Olney, John W., and Oi-Lan Ho. "Brain Damage in Infant Mice Following Oral Intake of Glutamate, Aspartate or Cysteine." *Nature* 227, no. 5258 (August 1970): 609–11. doi:10.1038/227609b0.

Olney, John W., Chandra H. Misra, and Vesa Rhee. "Brain and Retinal Damage from Lathyrus Excitotoxin, β-N-Oxalyl-L-α,β-Diaminopropionic Acid." *Nature* 264, no. 5587 (December 1976): 659–61. doi:10.1038/264659a0.

Olney, John W., Oi Lan Ho, and Vesela Rhee. "Brain-Damaging Potential of Protein Hydrolysates." *New England Journal of Medicine* 289, no. 8 (August 23, 1973): 391–95. doi:10.1056/nejm197308232890802.

Olney, John W., Theodore J. Cicero, Edward R. Meyer, and Tasia de Gubareff. "Acute Glutamate-Induced Elevations in Serum Testosterone and Luteinizing Hormone." *Brain Research* 112, no. 2 (August 1976): 420–24. doi:10.1016/0006-8993(76)90298-5.

Onaolapo, Adejoke Yetunde, and Olakunle James Onaolapo. "Glutamate and Depression: Reflecting a Deepening Knowledge of the Gut and Brain Effects of a Ubiquitous Molecule." *World Journal of Psychiatry* 11, no. 7 (July 19, 2021): 297–315. doi:10.5498/wjp.v11.i7.297.

Onaolapo, Olakunle James, Olaleye Samuel Aremu, and Adejoke Yetunde Onaolapo. "Monosodium Glutamate-Associated Alterations in Open Field, Anxiety-Related and Conditioned Place Preference Behaviours in Mice." *Naunyn-Schmiedeberg's Archives of Pharmacology* 390, no. 7 (March 29, 2017): 677–89. doi:10.1007/s00210-017-1371-6.

Oreskes, Naomi, and Erik M. Conway. *Merchants of Doubt: How a Handful of Scientists Obscured the Truth on Issues from Tobacco Smoke to Global Warming.* New York: Bloomsbury Publishing USA, 2010.

Ottosson, Filip, Einar Smith, Olle Melander, and Céline Fernandez. "Altered Asparagine and Glutamate Homeostasis Precede Coronary Artery Disease and Type 2 Diabetes." *Journal of Clinical Endocrinology & Metabolism* 103, no. 8 (May 16, 2018): 3060–69. doi:10.1210/jc.2018-00546.

Ottosson, Filip, Louise Brunkwall, Ulrika Ericson, Peter M. Nilsson, Peter Almgren, Céline Fernandez, Olle Melander, and Marju Orho-Melander. "Connection between BMI-Related Plasma Metabolite Profile and Gut Microbiota." *Journal of Clinical Endocrinology & Metabolism* 103, no. 4 (February 1, 2018): 1491–1501. doi:10.1210/jc.2017-02114.

Oya, Manami, Hideyuki Suzuki, Yuichiro Watanabe, Moritoshi Sato, and Takashi Tsuboi. "Amino Acid Taste Receptor Regulates Insulin Secretion in Pancreatic β-Cell Line MIN6 Cells." *Genes to Cells* 16, no. 5 (April 6, 2011): 608–16. doi:10.1111/j.1365-2443.2011.01509.x.

Pan American Health Organization. "Ultra-Processed Food and Drink Products in Latin America: Trends, Impact on Obesity, Policy Implications." Washington, DC: World Health Organization, 2015. https://iris.paho.org/bitstream/handle/10665.2/7699/9789275118641_eng.pdf.

Pasiakos, Stefan, Sanjiv Agarwal, Harris Lieberman, and Victor Fulgoni. "Sources and Amounts of Animal, Dairy, and Plant Protein Intake of US Adults in 2007–2010." *Nutrients* 7, no. 8 (August 21, 2015): 7058–69. doi:10.3390/nu7085322.

Pelsser, Lidy M., Klaas Frankena, Jan Toorman, Huub F. Savelkoul, Anthony E. Dubois, Rob Rodrigues Pereira, Ton A. Haagen, Nanda N. Rommelse, and Jan K. Buitelaar. "Effects of a Restricted Elimination Diet on the Behaviour of Children with Attention-Deficit Hyperactivity Disorder (INCA Study): A Randomised Controlled Trial." *The Lancet* 377, no. 9764 (February 2011): 494–503. doi:10.1016/s0140-6736(10)62227-1.

Perlmutter, David. *Drop Acid*. Hachette UK, 2022.

Pitt, David, Peter Werner, and Cedric S. Raine. "Glutamate Excitotoxicity in a Model of Multiple Sclerosis." *Nature Medicine* 6, no. 1 (January 2000): 67–70. doi:10.1038/71555.

Populin, T., S. Moret, S. Truant, and L. Conte. "A Survey on the Presence of Free Glutamic Acid in Foodstuffs, with and without Added Monosodium Glutamate." *Food Chemistry* 104, no. 4 (2007): 1712–17. doi:10.1016/j.foodchem.2007.03.034.

Port, Russell G., Lindsay M. Oberman, and Timothy P. L. Roberts. "Revisiting the Excitation/Inhibition Imbalance Hypothesis of ASD through a Clinical Lens." *British Journal of Radiology* 92, no. 1101 (September 2019): 20180944. doi:10.1259/bjr.20180944.

Prescott, John. "Effects of Added Glutamate on Liking for Novel Food Flavors." *Appetite* 42, no. 2 (April 2004): 143–50. doi:10.1016/j.appet.2003.08.013.

Prickett, T. D., and Y. Samuels. "Molecular Pathways: Dysregulated Glutamatergic Signaling Pathways in Cancer." *Clinical Cancer Research* 18, no. 16 (May 30, 2012): 4240–46. doi:10.1158/1078-0432.ccr-11-1217.

Purcell, A. E., O. H. Jeon, A. W. Zimmerman, M. E. Blue, and J. Pevsner. "Postmortem Brain Abnormalities of the Glutamate Neurotransmitter System in Autism." *Neurology* 57, no. 9 (November 13, 2001): 1618–28. doi:10.1212/wnl.57.9.1618.

Reid, Katherine. "Katie Reid and Smoothies for Health—Get Started Now." YouTube video, 2013. https://www.youtube.com/watch?v=4OsoDopmy1k.

Rico-Campà, Anaïs, Miguel A. Martínez-González, Ismael Alvarez-Alvarez, Raquel de Deus Mendonça, Carmen de la Fuente-Arrillaga, Clara Gómez-Donoso, and Maira Bes-Rastrollo. "Association between Consumption of Ultra-Processed Foods and All Cause Mortality: SUN Prospective Cohort Study." *BMJ* 365 (May 29, 2019): l1949. doi:10.1136/bmj.l1949.

Rigau, V., M. Morin, M.-C. Rousset, F. de Bock, A. Lebrun, P. Coubes, M.-C. Picot, et al. "Angiogenesis Is Associated with Blood-Brain Barrier Permeability in Temporal Lobe Epilepsy." *Brain* 130, no. 7 (May 29, 2007): 1942–56. doi:10.1093/brain/awm118.

Rogers, Michael D. "Further Studies Are Necessary in Order to Conclude a Causal Association between the Consumption of Monosodium L-Glutamate (MSG) and the Prevalence of Metabolic Syndrome in the Rural Thai Population." *Nutrition & Metabolism* 10, no. 1 (2013): 14. doi:10.1186/1743-7075-10-14.

Roosendaal, Stefan D., Kerstin Bendfeldt, Hugo Vrenken, Chris H. Polman, Stefan Borgwardt, Ernst W. Radue, Ludwig Kappos, et al. "Grey Matter Volume in a Large Cohort of MS Patients: Relation to MRI Parameters and Disability." *Multiple Sclerosis (Houndmills, Basingstoke, England)* 17, no. 9 (September 1, 2011): 1098–1106. doi:10.1177/1352458511404916.

Rosati, G. "The Prevalence of Multiple Sclerosis in the World: An Update." *Neurological Sciences* 22, no. 2 (April 1, 2001): 117–39. doi:10.1007/s100720170011.

Rowland, Ian, Glenn Gibson, Almut Heinken, Karen Scott, Jonathan Swann, Ines Thiele, and Kieran Tuohy. "Gut Microbiota Functions: Metabolism of Nutrients and Other Food Components." *European Journal of Nutrition* 57, no. 1 (April 9, 2017): 1–24. doi:10.1007/s00394-017-1445-8.

Rubenstein, J. L. R., and M. M. Merzenich. "Model of Autism: Increased Ratio of Excitation/Inhibition in Key Neural Systems." *Genes, Brain and Behavior* 2, no. 5 (October 16, 2003): 255–67. doi:10.1034/j.1601-183x.2003.00037.x.

Rudy, Carolyn C., Holly C. Hunsberger, Daniel S. Weitzner, and Miranda N. Reed. "The Role of the Tripartite Glutamatergic Synapse in the Pathophysiology of Alzheimer's Disease." *Aging and Disease* 6, no. 2 (2015): 131. doi:10.14336/ad.2014.0423.

Ruhl, A. "Glial Cells in the Gut." *Neurogastroenterology and Motility* 17, no. 6 (December 2005): 777–90. doi:10.1111/j.1365-2982.2005.00687.x.

Samuels, Adrienne. *The Man Who Sued the FDA.* Adrienne Samuels, 2013.

Samuels, Adrienne. *The Perfect Poison.* Adrienne Samuels, 2022.

Samuels, Adrienne. "The Toxicity/Safety of Processed Free Glutamic Acid (MSG): A Study in Suppression of Information." *Accountability in Research* 6, no. 4 (July 1999): 259–310. doi:10.1080/08989629908573933.

Sanacora, Gerard, Giulia Treccani, and Maurizio Popoli. "Towards a Glutamate Hypothesis of Depression." *Neuropharmacology* 62, no. 1 (January 2012): 63–77. doi:10.1016/j.neuropharm.2011.07.036.

Sand. J. "A Short History of MSG: Good Science, Bad Science, and Taste Cultures." *Gastronomica* 5, no. 4 (November 2005): 38–49. doi:10.1525/gfc.2005.5.4.38.

Sano, Chiaki. "History of Glutamate Production." *American Journal of Clinical Nutrition* 90, no. 3 (July 29, 2009): 728S732S. doi:10.3945 /ajcn.2009.27462f.

Savcheniuk, Oleksandr A., Oleksandr V. Virchenko, Tetyana M. Falalyeyeva, Tetyana V. Beregova, Lidia P. Babenko, Liudmyla M. Lazarenko, Olga M. Demchenko, Rostyslav V. Bubnov, and Mykola Ya Spivak. "The Efficacy of Probiotics for Monosodium Glutamate-Induced Obesity: Dietology Concerns and Opportunities for Prevention." *EPMA Journal* 5, no. 1 (January 13, 2014). doi:10.1186/1878-5085-5-2.

Savidge, Tor C., Michael V. Sofroniew, and Michel Neunlist. "Starring Roles for Astroglia in Barrier Pathologies of Gut and Brain." *Laboratory Investigation* 87, no. 8 (July 2, 2007): 731–36. doi:10.1038/labinvest.3700600.

Schmidt, Oliver I., Maria Morganti-Kossmann, Christoph E. Heyde, Daniel Perez, Ido Yatsiv, Esther Shohami, Wolfgang Ertel, and Philip F. Stahel. "Tumor Necrosis Factor-Mediated Inhibition of Interleukin-18 in the Brain: A Clinical and Experimental Study in Head-Injured Patients and in a Murine Model of Closed Head Injury." *Journal of Neuroinflammation* 1, no. 1 (2004): 13. doi:10.1186/1742-2094-1-13.

Schwartz, George R. *In Bad Taste: The MSG Symptom Complex: How Monosodium Glutamate Is a Major Cause of Treatable and Preventable Illnesses, such as Headaches, Asthma, Epilepsy, Heart Irregularities, Depression, Rage Reactions, and Attention Deficit Hyperactivity Disorder.* Santa Fe, NM: Health Press, 1999.

Scopp, Alfred L. "MSG and Hydrolyzed Vegetable Protein Induced Headache: Review and Case Studies." *Headache: The Journal of Head and Face Pain* 31, no. 2 (February 1991): 107–10. doi:10.1111/j.1526-4610.1991 .hed3102107.x.

Scrinis, Gyorgy, and Carlos Monteiro. "From Ultra-Processed Foods to Ultra-Processed Dietary Patterns." *Nature Food*, September 15, 2022. doi:10.1038 /s43016-022-00599-4.

Sharkey, Keith A., and Alfons B. A. Kroese. "Consequences of Intestinal Inflammation on the Enteric Nervous System: Neuronal Activation Induced by Inflammatory Mediators." *Anatomical Record* 262, no. 1 (January 1, 2001): 79–90. doi:10.1002/1097-0185(20010101)262:1<79::aid-ar1013>3.0.co;2-k.

Shell, Ellen Ruppel. "A New Theory of Obesity." *Scientific American*, October 2019. doi:10.1038/scientificamerican1019-38.

Sherwin, A., Y. Robitaille, F. Quesney, A. Olivier, J. Villemure, R. Leblanc, W. Feindel, et al. "Excitatory Amino Acids Are Elevated in Human Epileptic Cerebral Cortex." *Neurology* 38, no. 6 (June 1, 1988): 920–20. doi:10.1212 /wnl.38.6.920.

Shi, Zumin, Baojun Yuan, Anne W. Taylor, Yue Dai, Xiaoqun Pan, Tiffany K. Gill, and Gary A. Wittert. "Monosodium Glutamate Is Related to a Higher Increase in Blood Pressure over 5 Years: Findings from the Jiangsu Nutrition Study of Chinese Adults." *Journal of Hypertension* 29, no. 5 (May 2011): 846–53. doi:10.1097/hjh.0b013e328344da8e.

Shibuya, Ichiro, and Tetsuji Odani. "Method for Producing Amino-Acid-Rich Yeast." Google Patents, November 8, 2008. https://www.google.com/patents/EP2348100A1.

Siegel, Rebecca L., Kimberly D. Miller, and Ahmedin Jemal. "Cancer Statistics, 2019." *CA: A Cancer Journal for Clinicians* 69, no. 1 (January 2019): 7–34. doi:10.3322/caac.21551.

Siegel-Ramsay, Jennifer E., Liana Romaniuk, Heather C. Whalley, Neil Roberts, Holly Branigan, Andrew C. Stanfield, Stephen M. Lawrie, and Maria R. Dauvermann. "Glutamate and Functional Connectivity: Support for the Excitatory-Inhibitory Imbalance Hypothesis in Autism Spectrum Disorders." *Psychiatry Research: Neuroimaging* 313 (July 2021): 111302. doi:10.1016/j.pscychresns.2021.111302.

Skerry, Timothy M., and Paul G. Genever. "Glutamate Signalling in Non-Neuronal Tissues." *Trends in Pharmacological Sciences* 22, no. 4 (April 2001): 174–81. doi:10.1016/s0165-6147(00)01642-4.

Skurray, Geoffrey R., and Nicholas Pucar. "L-Glutamic Acid Content of Fresh and Processed Foods." *Food Chemistry* 27, no. 3 (January 1988): 177–80. doi:10.1016/0308-8146(88)90060-x.

Slimani, N., G. Deharveng, D. a. T. Southgate, C. Biessy, V. Chajès, M. M. E. van Bakel, M. C. Boutron-Ruault, et al. "Contribution of Highly Industrially Processed Foods to the Nutrient Intakes and Patterns of Middle-Aged Populations in the European Prospective Investigation into Cancer and Nutrition Study." *European Journal of Clinical Nutrition* 63, no. 4 (November 1, 2009): S206–S250. doi:10.1038/ejcn.2009.82.

Smith, Alan M., Marvin R. Natowicz, Daniel Braas, Michael A. Ludwig, Denise M. Ney, Elizabeth L. R. Donley, Robert E. Burrier, and David G. Amaral. "A Metabolomics Approach to Screening for Autism Risk in the Children's Autism Metabolome Project." *Autism Research* 13, no. 8 (June 18, 2020): 1270–85. doi:10.1002/aur.2330.

Smith, Jerry D., Chris M. Terpening, Siegfried O. F. Schmidt, and John G. Gums. "Relief of Fibromyalgia Symptoms Following Discontinuation of Dietary Excitotoxins." *Annals of Pharmacotherapy* 35, no. 6 (June 2001): 702–6. doi:10.1345/aph.10254.

Smith, Sarah L., and Edward D. Hall. "Mild Pre- and Posttraumatic Hypothermia Attenuates Blood-Brain Barrier Damage Following Controlled Cortical Impact Injury in the Rat." *Journal of Neurotrauma* 13, no. 1 (January 1996): 1–9. doi:10.1089/neu.1996.13.1.

Snitzer, Zach. "40M Americans Met Criteria for Substance Use Disorder in 2020: MARC." Maryland Addiction Recovery Center, November 1, 2021. https://www.marylandaddictionrecovery.com/40-million-americans -substance-use-disorder-2020/.

Sonnenburg, Justin, and Erica Sonnenburg. *The Good Gut.* Random House, 2015.

Stegink, L. D., G. L. Baker, and L. J. Filer. "Modulating Effect of Sustagen on Plasma Glutamate Concentration in Humans Ingesting Monosodium L-Glutamate." *American Journal of Clinical Nutrition* 37, no. 2 (February 1, 1983): 194–200. doi:10.1093/ajcn/37.2.194.

Stevens, Laura J., Thomas Kuczek, John R. Burgess, Elizabeth Hurt, and L. Eugene Arnold. "Dietary Sensitivities and ADHD Symptoms: Thirty-Five Years of Research." *Clinical Pediatrics* 50, no. 4 (December 2, 2010): 279–93. doi:10.1177/0009922810384728.

Substance Abuse and Mental Health Services Administration. "Results from the 2020 National Survey on Drug Use and Health: Detailed Tables," table 5.1A, Department of Health and Human Services, https://www.samhsa .gov/data/report/2020-nsduh-detailed-tables.

Takahashi, Nobuhiro, Takuichi Sato, and Tadashi Yamada. "Metabolic Pathways for Cytotoxic End Product Formation from Glutamate- and Aspartate-Containing Peptides by *Porphyromonas Gingivalis*." *Journal of Bacteriology* 182, no. 17 (September 2000): 4704–10. doi:10.1128/jb .182.17.4704-4710.2000.

Takano, Takahiro, Jane H.-C. Lin, Gregory Arcuino, Qun Gao, Jay Yang, and Maiken Nedergaard. "Glutamate Release Promotes Growth of Malignant Gliomas." *Nature Medicine* 7, no. 9 (September 1, 2001): 1010–15. doi:10.1038/nm0901-1010.

Taylor, Jill Bolte. *My Stroke of Insight: A Brain Scientist.* New York: Viking, 2006.

Teh, Jessica L. F., and Suzie Chen. "Glutamatergic Signaling in Cellular Transformation." *Pigment Cell & Melanoma Research* 25, no. 3 (February 20, 2012): 331–42. doi:10.1111/j.1755-148x.2012.00983.x.

Thiele, C., M. G. Gänzle, and R. F. Vogel. "Contribution of Sourdough Lactobacilli, Yeast, and Cereal Enzymes to the Generation of Amino Acids in Dough Relevant for Bread Flavor." *Cereal Chemistry Journal* 79, no. 1 (January 2002): 45–51. doi:10.1094/cchem.2002.79.1.45.

Torii, Kunio, Hisayuki Uneyama, and Eiji Nakamura. "Physiological Roles of Dietary Glutamate Signaling via Gut–Brain Axis Due to Efficient Digestion and Absorption." *Journal of Gastroenterology* 48, no. 4 (March 6, 2013): 442–51. doi:10.1007/s00535-013-0778-1.

Toyomasu, Yoshitaka, Erito Mochiki, Mitsuhiro Yanai, Kyoichi Ogata, Yuichi Tabe, Hiroyuki Ando, Tetsuro Ohno, Ryuusuke Aihara, Hiroaki Zai, and Hiroyuki Kuwano. "Intragastric Monosodium L-Glutamate Stimulates Motility of Upper Gut via Vagus Nerve in Conscious Dogs." *American Journal of Physiology-Regulatory, Integrative and Comparative Physiology* 298, no. 4 (April 2010): R1125–35. doi:10.1152/ajpregu.00691.2009.

Tripp, Gail, and Jeffery R. Wickens. "Neurobiology of ADHD." *Neuropharmacology* 57, no. 7–8 (December 2009): 579–89. doi:10.1016/j.neuropharm.2009.07.026.

TruthHurts315. "MSG on 60 Minutes (1991)."YouTube video, February 11, 2011. https://www.youtube.com/watch?v=8bwBfpWT1PU.

Tsuneyama, Koichi, Takeshi Nishida, Hayato Baba, Shu Taira, Makoto Fujimoto, Kazuhiro Nomoto, Shinichi Hayashi, et al. "Neonatal Monosodium Glutamate Treatment Causes Obesity, Diabetes, and Macrovesicular Steatohepatitis with Liver Nodules in DIAR Mice." *Journal of Gastroenterology and Hepatology* 29, no. 9 (August 25, 2014): 1736–43. doi:10.1111/jgh.12610.

Turnbaugh, Peter J., Micah Hamady, Tanya Yatsunenko, Brandi L. Cantarel, Alexis Duncan, Ruth E. Ley, Mitchell L. Sogin, et al. "A Core Gut Microbiome in Obese and Lean Twins." *Nature* 457, no. 7228 (November 30, 2008): 480–84. doi:10.1038/nature07540.

Turnbaugh, Peter J., Ruth E. Ley, Micah Hamady, Claire M. Fraser-Liggett, Rob Knight, and Jeffrey I. Gordon. "The Human Microbiome Project." *Nature* 449, no. 7164 (October 18, 2007): 804–10. doi:10.1038/nature06244.

U.S. Food and Drug Administration. "21CFR Part101 Food Labeling," 2008. https://www.govinfo.gov/content/pkg/CFR-2008-title21-vol2/xml/CFR -2008-title21-vol2-part101.xml.

U.S. Food and Drug Administration. "Questions and Answers on Monosodium Glutamate (MSG)." February 20, 2020. http://www.fda.gov /Food/IngredientsPackagingLabeling/FoodAdditivesIngredients/ucm 328728.htm.

Uno, Yota, and Joseph T. Coyle. "Glutamate Hypothesis in Schizophrenia." *Psychiatry and Clinical Neurosciences* 73, no. 5 (March 6, 2019): 204–15. doi:10.1111/pcn.12823.

Upadhyay, Huang, and R. J. Tamargo. "Inflammation in Stroke and Focal Cerebral Ischemia." *Surgical Neurology* 66, no. 3 (September 1, 2006): 232–45. doi:10.1016/j.surneu.2005.12.028.

Uys, Joachim D., and Kathryn J. Reissner. "Glutamatergic Neuroplasticity in Cocaine Addiction." *Progress in Molecular Biology and Translational Science* (2011): 367–400. doi:10.1016/b978-0-12-385506-0.00009-0.

Van der Kolk, Bessel, Mark Greenberg, Helene Boyd, and John Krystal. "Inescapable Shock, Neurotransmitters, and Addiction to Trauma: Toward a Psychobiology of Post Traumatic Stress." *Biological Psychiatry* 20, no. 3 (March 1985): 314–25. doi:https://doi.org/10.1016/0006-3223(85)90061-7.

Van Vliet, E. A, S. da Costa Araujo, S. Redeker, R. van Schaik, E. Aronica, and J. A. Gorter. "Blood-Brain Barrier Leakage May Lead to Progression of Temporal Lobe Epilepsy." *Brain* 130, no. 2 (February 1, 2007): 521–34. doi:10.1093/brain/awl318.

Velasquez-Manoff, Moises. *An Epidemic of Absence : A New Way of Understanding Allergies and Autoimmune Diseases.* New York, Ny: Scribner, 2013.

Ventura, Alison K., Gary K. Beauchamp, and Julie A. Mennella. "Infant Regulation of Intake: The Effect of Free Glutamate Content in Infant Formulas." *American Journal of Clinical Nutrition* 95, no. 4 (February 22, 2012): 875–81. doi:10.3945/ajcn.111.024919.

Wahls, Terry, Maria O. Scott, Zaidoon Alshare, Linda Rubenstein, Warren Darling, Lucas Carr, Karen Smith, Catherine A. Chenard, Nicholas LaRocca, and Linda Snetselaar. "Dietary Approaches to Treat MS-Related Fatigue: Comparing the Modified Paleolithic (Wahls Elimination) and Low Saturated Fat (Swank) Diets on Perceived Fatigue in Persons with Relapsing-Remitting Multiple Sclerosis: Study Protocol for a Randomized Controlled Trial." *Trials* 19 (June 4, 2018). doi:10.1186/s13063-018-2680-x.

Walker, A. K., A. Kavelaars, C. J. Heijnen, and R. Dantzer. "Neuroinflammation and Comorbidity of Pain and Depression." *Pharmacological Reviews* 66, no. 1 (December 11, 2013): 80–101. doi:10.1124/pr.113.008144.

Wang, Guo-Du, Xi-Yu Wang, Yun Xia, and Jackie D. Wood. "Dietary Glutamate: Interactions with the Enteric Nervous System." *Journal of Neurogastroenterology and Motility* 20, no. 1 (January 31, 2014): 41–53. doi:10.5056/jnm.2014.20.1.41.

Wang, Ji, Fushun Wang, Dongmei Mai, and Shaogang Qu. "Molecular Mechanisms of Glutamate Toxicity in Parkinson's Disease." *Frontiers in Neuroscience* 14 (November 26, 2020). doi:10.3389/fnins.2020.585584.

Wang, Lu, Mengxi Du, Kai Wang, Neha Khandpur, Sinara Laurini Rossato, Jean-Philippe Drouin-Chartier, Euridice Martínez Steele, Edward Giovannucci, Mingyang Song, and Fang Fang Zhang. "Association of Ultra-Processed Food Consumption with Colorectal Cancer Risk among Men and Women: Results from Three Prospective US Cohort Studies." *BMJ* 378 (August 31, 2022): e068921. doi:10.1136/bmj-2021-068921.

Weissberg, Itai, Aljoscha Reichert, Uwe Heinemann, and Alon Friedman. "Blood-Brain Barrier Dysfunction in Epileptogenesis of the Temporal Lobe." *Epilepsy Research and Treatment* 2011 (June 7, 2011): 1–10. doi:10.1155/2011/143908.

Wieseler-Frank, Julie, Steven F. Maier, and Linda R. Watkins. "Glial Activation and Pathological Pain." *Neurochemistry International* 45, no. 2–3 (2004): 389–95. Doi:10.1016/j.neuint.2003.09.009.

Xavier, R. J., and D. K. Podolsky. "Unravelling the Pathogenesis of Inflammatory Bowel Disease." *Nature* 448, no. 7152 (July 2007): 427–34. Doi:10.1038/nature06005.

Yang, Pinchen, and Chen-Lin Chang. "Glutamate-Mediated Signaling and Autism Spectrum Disorders: Emerging Treatment Targets." *Current Pharmaceutical Design* 20, no. 32 (January 10, 2014): 5186–93. Doi:10.217 4/13816128196661401101120725.

Yang, Wenhan, Ru Yang, Jing Luo, Lei He, Jun Liu, and Jun Zhang. "Increased Absolute Glutamate Concentrations and Glutamate-to-Creatine Ratios in Patients with Methamphetamine Use Disorders." *Frontiers in Psychiatry* 9 (August 31, 2018). doi:10.3389/fpsyt.2018.00368.

Yolken, R. H., and E. F. Torrey. "Are Some Cases of Psychosis Caused by Microbial Agents? A Review of the Evidence." *Molecular Psychiatry* 13, no. 5 (May 1, 2008): 470–79. doi:10.1038/mp.2008.5.

Yong, Ed. *I Contain Multitudes: The Microbes within Us and a Grander View of Life*. New York: Ecco, 2018.

Zolotarev, Vasiliy, Raisa Khropycheva, Hisayuki Uneyama, and Kunio Torii. "Effect of Free Dietary Glutamate on Gastric Secretion in Dogs." *Annals of the New York Academy of Sciences* 1170, no. 1 (July 2009): 87–90. doi:10.1111/j.1749-6632.2009.03900.x.

INDEX

ABOUT THE AUTHORS

Katherine Reid, PhD, is a biochemist and the founder of Unblind My Mind, Inc., a non-profit 501(c)(3) organization dedicated to improving health through informed food choices. Previously she worked in the Silicon Valley biotech industry in the development of cancer pharmaceuticals and diagnostics. Today she works with individuals and families in collaboration with the medical and biotech communities to devise data-driven food solutions for chronic inflammatory illnesses. She lives with her family in the Santa Cruz mountains.

Barbara Price, MS, MA, PhD, has studied topics ranging from climate change to protein biophysics and has turned her passion for science into a career as a science writer and editor. As a senior science development editor for major educational publishers, she helps textbook authors turn highly technical information into narratives that teach. As an editor and science writer, she supports scientists who have their own stories to tell. Price has also authored original content for young learners and general audiences. She lives in Northern California.